THE NEXT GENERATION OF
BIOMEDICAL AND BEHAVIORAL
SCIENCES RESEARCHERS

Breaking Through

Ronald Daniels and Lida Beninson, *Editors*

Committee on the Next Generation Initiative

Board on Higher Education and Workforce

Policy and Global Affairs

A Consensus Study Report of

The National Academies of
SCIENCES • ENGINEERING • MEDICINE

THE NATIONAL ACADEMIES PRESS
Washington, DC
www.nap.edu

THE NATIONAL ACADEMIES PRESS   500 Fifth Street, NW   Washington, DC 20001

This activity was supported by contracts between the National Academy of Sciences and The National Institutes of Health (#HHSN263201200074I, Order No. HHSN26300107) and the Bloomberg Philanthropies. Any opinions, findings, conclusions, or recommendations expressed in this publication do not necessarily reflect the views of any organization or agency that provided support for the project.

International Standard Book Number-13: 978-0-309-47137-4
International Standard Book Number-10: 0-309-47137-0
Library of Congress Control Number 2018941722
Digital Object Identifier: https://doi.org/10.17226/25008

Additional copies of this publication are available for sale from the National Academies Press, 500 Fifth Street, NW, Keck 360, Washington, DC 20001; (800) 624-6242 or (202) 334-3313; http://www.nap.edu.

Copyright 2018 by the National Academy of Sciences. All rights reserved.

Printed in the United States of America

Suggested citation: National Academies of Sciences, Engineering, and Medicine. 2018. *The Next Generation of Biomedical and Behavioral Sciences Researchers: Breaking Through*. Washington, DC: The National Academies Press. doi: https://doi.org/10.17226/25008.

The National Academies of
SCIENCES · ENGINEERING · MEDICINE

The **National Academy of Sciences** was established in 1863 by an Act of Congress, signed by President Lincoln, as a private, nongovernmental institution to advise the nation on issues related to science and technology. Members are elected by their peers for outstanding contributions to research. Dr. Marcia McNutt is president.

The **National Academy of Engineering** was established in 1964 under the charter of the National Academy of Sciences to bring the practices of engineering to advising the nation. Members are elected by their peers for extraordinary contributions to engineering. Dr. C. D. Mote, Jr., is president.

The **National Academy of Medicine** (formerly the Institute of Medicine) was established in 1970 under the charter of the National Academy of Sciences to advise the nation on medical and health issues. Members are elected by their peers for distinguished contributions to medicine and health. Dr. Victor J. Dzau is president.

The three Academies work together as the **National Academies of Sciences, Engineering, and Medicine** to provide independent, objective analysis and advice to the nation and conduct other activities to solve complex problems and inform public policy decisions. The National Academies also encourage education and research, recognize outstanding contributions to knowledge, and increase public understanding in matters of science, engineering, and medicine.

Learn more about the National Academies of Sciences, Engineering, and Medicine at www.nationalacademies.org.

The National Academies of
SCIENCES • ENGINEERING • MEDICINE

Consensus Study Reports published by the National Academies of Sciences, Engineering, and Medicine document the evidence-based consensus on the study's statement of task by an authoring committee of experts. Reports typically include findings, conclusions, and recommendations based on information gathered by the committee and the committee's deliberations. Each report has been subjected to a rigorous and independent peer-review process and it represents the position of the National Academies on the statement of task.

Proceedings published by the National Academies of Sciences, Engineering, and Medicine chronicle the presentations and discussions at a workshop, symposium, or other event convened by the National Academies. The statements and opinions contained in proceedings are those of the participants and are not endorsed by other participants, the planning committee, or the National Academies.

For information about other products and activities of the National Academies, please visit www.nationalacademies.org/about/whatwedo.

COMMITTEE ON THE NEXT GENERATION INITIATIVE

Members

RONALD J. DANIELS (*Chair*), President, Johns Hopkins University
NANCY C. ANDREWS (NAS/NAM), Dean and Vice Chancellor for Academic Affairs (Emerita), Duke University School of Medicine
W. TRAVIS BERGGREN, Founding Director for the Stem Cell Research Core Facility, Salk Institute
SUE BIGGINS (NAS), Associate Director in the Division of Basic Sciences, Fred Hutchinson Cancer Research Center, Investigator, Howard Hughes Medical Institute
JOHN BOOTHROYD (NAS), Burt and Marion Avery Professor, Department of Microbiology and Immunology, Associate Vice Provost for Graduate Education, Stanford University
DAVID R. BURGESS, Professor of Biology, Boston College
KAFUI DZIRASA, Assistant Professor of Psychiatry and Behavioral Sciences, Duke University
GIOVANNA GUERRERO-MEDINA, Executive Director, Ciencia Puerto Rico; Director, Yale Ciencia Initiative, Yale University
JUDITH KIMBLE (NAS), Vilas Professor in the Department of Biochemistry, University of Wisconsin-Madison, Investigator, Howard Hughes Medical Institute
STORY LANDIS (NAM), Former Director of the National Institute of Neurological Disorders and Stroke, National Institutes of Health
KENNETH MAYNARD, Head, Global Patient Safety Evaluation (GPSE) Compliance, Standards and Training and GPSE Business Partners Relations, Takeda Pharmaceuticals International Co.
GARY S. MCDOWELL, Executive Director, The Future of Research, Inc.
JESSICA POLKA, Visiting Scholar, Whitehead Institute
JOAN Y. REEDE (NAM), Dean for Diversity and Community Partnership and Professor of Medicine, Harvard Medical School
LANA R. SKIRBOLL, Vice President of Science Policy, Sanofi
PAULA STEPHAN, Professor of Economics, Georgia State University
MARIA ELENA ZAVALA, Professor of Biology, California State University, Northridge

Study Staff

LIDA BENINSON, Study Director and Program Officer, Board on Higher Education and Workforce
MARIA LUND DAHLBERG, Program Officer
YASMEEN HUSSAIN, Associate Program Officer (*Until July 2017*)

ELIZABETH GARBEE, Christine Mirzayan Science and Technology Policy Graduate Fellow (*Until April 2018*)
AUSTEN APPLEGATE, Senior Program Assistant
LAYNE SCHERER, Program Officer
JAY LABOV, Senior Advisor for Education and Communication
IRENE NGUN, Research Associate
ADRIANA COUREMBIS, Finance Officer
ALLISON BERGER, Senior Program Assistant
FREDRICK LESTINA, Senior Program Assistant
JAIME COLMAN, Senior Program Assistant (*Until December 2017*)
THOMAS RUDIN, Director, Board on Higher Education and Workforce

Consultants

JOE ALPER, Writer
JEREMY BERG, Consultant
PHILLIP SPECTOR, Consultant

BOARD ON HIGHER EDUCATION AND WORKFORCE

Members

RICHARD K. MILLER (*Chair*) (NAE), President, Olin College of Engineering
LAWRENCE D. BOBO (NAS), W.E.B. Du Bois Professor of the Social Sciences, Department of Sociology, Harvard University
ANGELA BYARS-WINSTON, Professor of Medicine, University of Wisconsin–Madison
JAIME CURTIS-FISK, Scientist and STEM Education Program Leader, The Dow Chemical Company
APRILLE ERICSSON, Capture–Mission Manager, NASA Goddard Space Flight Center
RICHARD FREEMAN, Herbert Ascherman Professor of Economics, Harvard University
PAUL J. LEBLANC, President, Southern New Hampshire University
SALLY F. MASON, President Emerita, University of Iowa
FRANCISCO RODRIGUEZ, Chancellor, Los Angeles Community College District
SUBHASH SINGHAL (NAE), Battelle Fellow Emeritus, Pacific Northwest National Laboratory
KUMBLE R. SUBBASWAMY, Chancellor, University of Massachusetts, Amherst
SHELLEY WESTMAN, Principal/Partner, Ernst & Young, LLP
MARY WOOLLEY (NAM), President and CEO, Research! America

Staff

AUSTEN APPLEGATE, Senior Program Assistant
ASHLEY BEAR, Program Officer
LIDA BENINSON, Program Officer
ALLISON BERGER, Senior Program Assistant
JAIME COLMAN, Senior Program Assistant (*Until December, 2017*)
MARIA LUND DAHLBERG, Program Officer
YASMEEN HUSSAIN, Associate Program Officer (*Until July 2017*)
LEIGH JACKSON, Senior Program Officer
FREDRICK LESTINA, Senior Program Assistant
BARBARA NATALIZIO, Program Officer
IRENE NGUN, Research Associate
LAYNE SCHERER, Program Officer
THOMAS RUDIN, Director

Preface

The U.S. biomedical research ecosystem is one of the great engines of innovation in modern history. It is a wellspring of discovery and cures that has expanded the domain of human knowledge, improved and saved countless lives, and catalyzed job growth and economic prosperity in communities across the nation. The United States' model for training and funding the biomedical workforce is widely credited with making it a global leader in scientific research, one that is emulated around the world. But there is nothing inevitable about the success of this enterprise. It requires constant vigilance and stewardship, to ensure that we are setting the optimal conditions and incentives for our scientists and the science they imagine, now and into the future.

There have been warning signs for years that the enterprise may be calcifying—in ways that create barriers, in particular for the incoming generation of researchers. Multiple national reports have been penned about these warning signs, and they have proposed countless recommendations for reform. But many of the recommendations have gone unaddressed. And the problems have endured.

Of late, the vulnerabilities in the biomedical enterprise have grown more evident, leading to renewed concern on the part of science policy leaders, professional organizations, funding agencies, and, above all, the U.S. Congress, which called on the National Academy of Sciences to conduct a comprehensive study of the policies affecting the next generation of researchers in the United States. This report is the outcome of that study. In developing it, we saw our task as two-fold: First, to identify reforms that are tailored to the evolving barriers facing the next generation of researchers. But, second, to do so in a manner that responds to the failure of many of the earlier recommendations to gain traction.

The pages that follow chronicle a biomedical research landscape of remarkable promise, yet characterized by fissures and areas of stress. This report offers a set of recommendations that seek to engage those vulnerabilities and to build an ecosystem that is dynamic and fair, while setting in place the structures and conditions for sustained change, so that episodic reports start to fall away and policy change across the enterprise is ongoing and enduring, to benefit the next generation of researchers, as well as the generations of researchers yet to come.

>Ronald Daniels, Chair
>Committee on the Next Generation Initiative

Acknowledgments

The committee would like to acknowledge the National Institutes of Health (NIH) and Bloomberg Philanthropies for their generous support of this study. In particular, the committee would like to acknowledge Phillip Spector, Yasmeen Hussain, and Amanda Field for their support to this project. The committee also acknowledges the contributions from Walter Schaffer, Jennifer Sutton, Silda Nikaj, Katrina Pearson, Deepshikha Roychowdhury, and Robert Moore of NIH for their support and responses to data requests. The committee would also like to acknowledge the University of California, San Francisco, The Johns Hopkins University, and Sanofi in Cambridge, Massachusetts, for hosting the committee's meetings. We are also grateful for the contributions of James Burke, Gilbert S. Omenn Fellow at the National Academy of Medicine; Rona Briere, for her careful editing of the report; and Rebecca Morgan of the National Academies Research Center, for her assistance with fact-checking.

ACKNOWLEDGMENT OF PRESENTERS

The committee gratefully acknowledges the contributions of the following individuals:

DAVID ASAI, Senior Director for Science Education, Howard Hughes Medical Institute
ELIZABETH BACA, Senior Health Advisor, California Governor's Office of Planning and Research
SUSAN BASERGA, Professor of Molecular Biophysics and Biochemistry, Yale University

MARC BONNEFOI, Head, R&D France, Sanofi
GWYNETH CARD, Group Leader, Howard Hughes Medical Institute, Janelia Research Center
DENNIS DEAN, II, R&D Scientist, Seven Bridges Genomics
DEBORAH DUNSIRE, CEO, XTuit Pharmaceuticals
KENNETH GIBBS, Program Director, Division of Training, Workforce Development, and Diversity, National Institute of General Medicine, National Institutes of Health
RORY GOODWIN, Neurosurgery Resident, The Johns Hopkins University Hospital
EVA GUINAN, Director of Translational Research, Radiation Oncology, Dana-Farber Cancer Institute
STEPHEN HAGGARTY, Associate Professor of Neurology, Harvard Medical School, Director, Chemical Neurobiology Laboratory, Center for Genomic Medicine, Massachusetts General Hospital
MISTY HEGGENESS, Chief of Longitudinal Research, Evaluation, and Outreach, U.S. Census Bureau
SAMANTHA HINDLE, Assistant Professional Researcher, University of California, San Francisco
STEVEN HYMAN, Distinguished Service Professor, Harvard University, Director, Stanley Center for Psychiatric Research, Core Member, Broad Institute
BAHIJA JALLAL, Executive Vice President, MedImmune
MARC KIRSCHNER, John Franklin Enders University Professor, Chair, Department of Systems Biology, Harvard Medical School
MICHAEL LAUER, Director, Office of Extramural Research, National Institutes of Health
ALAN LESHNER, CEO Emeritus, American Association for the Advancement of Science
KAY LUND, Director of the Division of Biomedical Research Workforce, Office of Extramural Research, National Institutes of Health
TERRY MAGNUSON, Vice Chancellor for Research, University of North Carolina at Chapel Hill
SEAN MCCONNELL, Postdoctoral Scholar, University of Chicago
PAUL MCGONIGLE, Director, Interdisciplinary & Career-Oriented Programs, Co-Director, Drug Discovery & Development Program, Drexel University
JIM MULLEN, CEO, Patheon
MARINA RAMON, Board of Directors, National Postdoctoral Association
MICHAEL RICHEY, Associate Technical Fellow, Learning Sciences and Engineering Education Research, The Boeing Company
LAWRENCE ROTHBLUM, Chair of the Department of Cell Biology, University of Oklahoma, President, Association of Anatomy, Cell Biology and Neurobiology Chairpersons

NANCY SCHWARTZ, Professor, Department of Biomedical Sciences, University of Chicago
SHIRLEY TILGHMAN, President of the University, Emeritus, Professor of Molecular Biology and Public Affairs, Princeton University
DANIEL WILSON, Research Advisor, Economic Research Department, Federal Reserve Bank of San Francisco

ACKNOWLEDGMENT OF REVIEWERS

This Consensus Study Report was reviewed in draft form by individuals chosen for their diverse perspectives and technical expertise. The purpose of this independent review is to provide candid and critical comments that will assist the National Academies of Sciences, Engineering, and Medicine in making its published report as sound as possible and to ensure that the report meets institutional standards for objectivity, evidence, and responsiveness to the study charge. The review comments and draft manuscript remain confidential to protect the integrity of the process.

We wish to thank the following individuals for their review of this report: Bruce Alberts, University of California, San Francisco; Georges Benjamin, American Public Health Association; Sherilynn Black, Duke University; Gregory Burke, Wake Forest University; John Burris, Burroughs Wellcome Fund; Deborah Dunsire, Xtuit Pharmaceuticals; Samantha Hindle, University of California, San Francisco; Timothy Ley, Washington University, St. Louis; Ross McKinney, Association of American Medical Colleges; Christopher Pickett, Rescuing Biomedical Research; Therese Richmond, University of Pennsylvania; Sally Rockey, Foundation for Food and Agriculture Research; Lawrence Rothblum, University of Oklahoma; Henry Sauermann, European School of Management and Technology, Berlin; Geoffrey Smith, Digitalis Ventures; and Wayne Yokoyama, Washington University, St. Louis.

Although the reviewers listed above have provided many constructive comments and suggestions, they were not asked to endorse the conclusions or recommendations, nor did they see the final draft of the report before its release. The review of this report was overseen by Olufunmilayo (Funmi) Olopade, University of Chicago and Charles Phelps, University of Rochester. They were responsible for making certain that an independent examination of this report was carried out in accordance with the standards of the National Academies and that all review comments were carefully considered. Responsibility for the final content rests entirely with the authoring committee and the National Academies.

Contents

BOXES AND FIGURES — xvii

ACRONYMS AND ABBREVIATIONS — xix

SUMMARY — 1

1 INTRODUCTION AND OVERVIEW — 13
   Work of the Committee, 14
   Scope of the Study, 16
   Structure of the Report, 17
   Reference, 17

2 THE LANDSCAPE FOR THE NEXT GENERATION OF RESEARCHERS — 19
   Doctoral and Medical Training in Biomedical Research, 19
   The Postdoctoral Research Experience, 21
   Transition to Independent Research Postitions, 27
   Funding for an Independent Research Career, 32
   Other Challenges in Pursuing Research Careers, 42
   References, 45

3 TRANSPARENCY, SHARED RESPONSIBILITY, AND SUSTAINABILITY — 49
   Shared Responsibility, 49
   Increasing Diversity and Inclusion, 53

Increasing Transparency, 55
Sustainability, 60
References, 63

4 TRANSITIONING TO INDEPENDENCE 65
Training and Support for All Postdoctoral Researchers, 66
Optimizing the Duration and Support Mechanisms for Postdoctoral Training, 70
Create Opportunities for Entrepreneurial Activity, 77
References, 79

5 BUILDING A BETTER ECOSYSTEM FOR INDEPENDENCE 81
References, 92

6 EXPERIMENTATION AND INNOVATION 95
References, 99

7 FINAL THOUGHTS AND SUMMARY OF RECOMMENDATIONS BY ACTOR 101
The Recommendations—By Stakeholder, 102

APPENDIXES

A Definitions Used in the Report 107
B Responses to Recommendations in Previous Reports on Biomedical and Behavioral Researchers 109
C Dear Colleague Letter 145
D Committee Member Biographies 153
E Committee Meeting Agendas 163

Boxes and Figures

BOXES

1-1   Statement of Task, 15

2-1   Postdoctoral Researcher: 2018 Definitions and Characterizations, 22

3-1   NSF Data Surveys, 59

FIGURES

2-1   Percentage of U.S. trained biomedical individuals living in the United States, sector of employment by cohort and position, 1993-2013, 28
2-2   Proportion of NIH research project grant direct cost dollars awarded by age group, 30
2-3   NIH appropriations in current and constant dollars, 1995-2017, 33
2-4   Success rates for competing type 1 R01 success rates for new and established investigators, 33
2-5   Individual applicants, awardees, and funding rates of NIH research project grants, 35
2-6   Number of investigators supported by NIH R01-equivalent awards by career stage, 36
2-7   Age at first-R01 equivalent by degree type, 37
2-8   Years to first R01-equivalent award since last degree award, 38
2-9   Average age over time to first R01, new (type 1) second R01, and renewal (type 2) second R01, 38
2-10 Age at first R01-equivalent award by NIH Institute, 39

xvii

2-11 First competing research project grant award received by investigators, 41
2-12 Academic science and engineering research and development expenditures, by source of funding, 43
2-13 Dropout of first-time R01-funded NIH investigators, 44

B-1 Trends in the K99 research career development award: Competing applications and awards between 2007 and 2016, 114
B-2 Trends in F32 awards: The success rate for F32 applications by degree between 2011 and 2016, 115
B-3 Trends in F32 applications: Numbers of competing applications (top left: all applicants; top right: medical degree-holding applicants only) and percent of applicants with particular degrees (bottom: all applicants) between 2007 and 2016, 116
B-4 Trends in NRSA awards: (top) Competing applications, awards, and success rates between 1998 and 2016 for F32 postdoctoral fellowships; (bottom) Awarded NRSA training and fellowship positions by pre-doctoral and postdoctoral status between 1998 and 2016, 118
B-5 Trends in T32 awards: Number of awards between 2007 and 2016, 119
B-6 NRSA postdoctoral salaries in nominal and constant dollars. Left: in constant 1975 and 2012 dollars since 1975; Right: in 2012 dollars since 2011, 121
B-7 Survey of health benefits for postdoctoral researchers, 123
B-8 Success rates for new (type1) R01-equivalent grants, by career stage of investigator, 135
B-9 Number of investigators supported on competing research project grants, by career stage of investigator, 135

Acronyms and Abbreviations

AAAS	American Association for the Advancement of Science
AAMC	Association of American Medical Colleges
AAU	Association of American Universities
ACD	Advisory Committee to the NIH Director
AMGDB	Association of Medical and Graduate Departments of Biochemistry
ARRA	American Recovery Reinvestment Act
ASBMB	American Society for Biochemistry and Molecular Biology
ASCB	American Society for Cell Biology
B.A.	Bachelor of Arts
BEST	Broadening Experiences in Scientific Training
BHEW	Board on Higher Education and Workforce
BLS	Bureau of Labor Statistics
BRAINS	Biobehavioral Research Awards for Innovative New Scientists
BRAINS	Brain Research through Advancing Innovative Neurotechnologies
BRAINS	Broadening the Representation of Academic Investigators in Neuroscience
BREC	Biomedical Research Enterprise Council
B.S.	Bachelor of Science
BUILD	Building Infrastructure Leading to Diversity
CEC	Coordination and Evaluation Center
CFR	Code of Federal Regulations
CGS	Council of Graduate Schools

COMPASS	Committee for Postdocs and Students
COSEMPUP	Committee for Science, Engineering, Medicine, and Public Policy
COSWD	Chief Officer for Scientific Workforce Diversity
CPI	Consumer Price Index
CSR	Center for Scientific Review
CTSA	Clinical Translational Science Awards
DICP	Harvard Medical School's Office for Diversity Inclusion and Community Partnership
DLR	Division of Loan Repayment at NIH
DPC	NIH Diversity Program Consortium
EEI	Early Established Investigator
ESI	Early-Stage Investigator
FASEB	Federation of Societies for Experimental Biology
FLSA	Fair Labor Standards Act
FRLC	Future Research Leaders Conference
FY	Fiscal Year
HHMI	Howard Hughes Medical Institute
HHS	U.S. Department of Health and Human Services
HMS	Harvard Medical School
ICs	Institutes and Centers
IDP	Individual Development Plan
IPUMS	Integrated Public Use Microdata Series
IRACDA	Institutional Research and Academic Career Development Award
IRIS	Institute for Research on Innovation and Science
LPR	Loan Repayment Program
LRP	Loan Repayment Award
MARC/RISE	Maximizing Access to Research Careers (MARC) and Research Initiative for Scientific Enhancement
M.B.A.	Master's of Business Administration
M.D.	Medical Doctorate
MERIT	Method to Extend Research in Time
MIRA	Maximizing Investigators' Research Award
MIT	Massachusetts Institute of Technology
M.S.	Master of Science

NAS	National Academy of Sciences
NCI	National Cancer Institute
NEI	National Eye Institute
NGRI	Next Generation Researchers Initiative
NGRI-DS	Next Generation Researchers Initiative Diversity Supplements
NHLBI	National Heart, Lung, and Blood Institute
NIAID	National Institute of Allergy and Infectious Diseases
NIBIB	National Institute of Biomedical Imaging and Engineering
NIDCR	National Institute of Dental and Craniofacial Research
NIDDK	National Institute of Diabetes and Digestive and Kidney Diseases
NIGMS	National Institute of General Medical Sciences
NIH	National Institutes of Health
NIMH	National Institute of Mental Health
NINDS	National Institute for Neurological Disorders and Stroke
NPA	National Postdoctoral Association
NRC	National Research Council
NRMN	National Research Mentoring Network
NRSA	Ruth L. Kirschstein National Research Service Award
NSCG	National Survey of College Graduates
NSERC	National Science and Engineering Research Council
NSF	National Science Foundation
NSF ADVANCE	National Science Foundation Increasing the Participation and Advancement of Women in Academic Science and Engineering Careers
NSF GRP	National Science Foundation Graduate Research Program
NSRCG	National Survey of Recent College Graduates
ORCID	Open Researcher and Contributor Identification
PD/PI	Program Director/Principal Investigator
Ph.D.	Doctorate of Philosophy
PI	Principle Investigator
R&D	Research and Development
RBR	Rescuing Biomedical Research
RPG	Research Project Grant
RPPR	Research Performance Progress Report
S&E	Science and Engineering
SACNAS	Society for the Advancement of Chicanos/Hispanics and Native Americans in Science
SBIR	Small Business Innovation Research

SDR	Survey on Doctoral Recipients
STEM	Science, Technology, Engineering, and Mathematics
STTR	Small Business Technology Transfer
SWD	Scientific Workforce Diversity
UCSF	University of California, San Francisco
UIDP	University Industry Demonstration Partnership
UMBC	University of Maryland Baltimore County
URM	Underrepresented Minority

Summary

Since the end of the Second World War, the United States has developed the world's preeminent system for biomedical[1] research, one that has given rise to revolutionary medical advances as well as a dynamic and innovative business sector generating high-quality jobs and powering economic output and exports for the U.S. economy. Although the United States remains the global leader in science and technology, measured in terms of the funding level, number of scientists supported, discoveries made, awards received, industries supported, and impacts on the quality of health, the U.S. global share of science and technology activities is waning as that of other nations, especially China, continues to rise (National Science Board, 2018). Indeed, there is a growing concern that the biomedical research enterprise, for all of its many strengths, is beset by several core challenges that undercut its vitality, promise, and productivity and that could diminish its critical role in the nation's health and innovation in the biomedical industry.

Among the most salient of these challenges is the gulf between the burgeoning number of scientists qualified to participate in this system as academic researchers and the elusive opportunities to establish long-term research careers in academia. One measure of initial career success is obtaining a tenure-track research position. In 1973, 55 percent of Ph.D.'s in the biological sciences received a tenure-track academic research position within 6 years, compared to 18 percent in 2009 (Cyranoski et al., 2011). Meanwhile, a decline in research funding in real dollars, combined with broader demographic trends, has reduced success rates for grant applications, and the average age of first receipt of a major

---

[1] In this report, "biomedical" refers to the full range of biological, biomedical, behavioral, and health sciences supported by the National Institutes of Health.

National Institutes of Health (NIH) independent grant, the R01, has risen from 36 years in 1980 to 43 years in 2016.[2] Those investigators who do secure an R01 or equivalent NIH grant face increasing pressure to secure additional sources of research funding to prevent the closure of their laboratories if their grant is not renewed. Additionally, women and underrepresented minorities face persistent and endemic obstacles to success in securing tenure-track faculty positions and advancing through the professoriate.

Another set of issues affecting the future of the biomedical workforce concerns the nature of the training young scientists receive, and the mismatch between that training and their career prospects. The focus of young scientists on securing an academic research faculty position can lead them to overlook opportunities as independent researchers in other areas, such as in start-up and established industries, foundations, and government. Significantly, these opportunities may require training experiences different from those associated with traditional academic careers. Yet too many postdoctoral researchers pursue training experiences with the objective of later securing an academic position, rather than enhancing their ability to compete for the range of fulfilling, independent careers that exist outside of academia, where the majority will be employed.

At the same time, there is concern that too many newly awarded biomedical Ph.D., M.D., and M.D.-Ph.D. holders spend prolonged periods in postdoctoral positions[3] currently characterized by low salaries, inadequate training and mentorship, and few opportunities for independent research or professional advancement. Although some individuals take postdoctoral positions because they are unsure of which career path to pursue or because they believe postdoctoral experience is necessary to obtain a position in sectors outside of academia, many linger as postdoctoral researchers as they wait for academic research positions to open. In the near future, it is likely that the number of Ph.D.-level researchers entering the system will exceed the number of faculty research positions available to them. Although young scientists certainly have the right to compete for the positions they desire, they must do so with a realistic understanding of their career prospects and, as much as possible, be encouraged to explore other career options sooner rather than spending time in long or multiple postdoctoral positions.

These obstacles to success have created a research career path that is increasingly unattractive, in terms of pay, duration, culture, risk-taking, and future job

---

[2] See https://grants.nih.gov/grants/new_investigators/Age_Degree-First-Time-117-16_RFM_lls_25march2016_DR-Approved.xlsx (accessed February 17, 2018).

[3] Several definitions of a postdoctoral researcher are listed in Chapter 2, but this report uses the NIH Office of Intramural Training and Education's definition: "A postdoc is an individual with a doctoral degree (PhD, MD, DDS, or the equivalent) who is engaged in a temporary period of mentored research and/or scholarly training for the purpose of acquiring the professional skills needed to pursue a career path of his or her choosing." See https://www.training.nih.gov/resources/faqs/postdoc_irp (accessed February 2, 2018).

prospects, as well as an environment in which scientific misconduct appears to be increasing (Edwards and Roy, 2017). As the National Academies *Bridges to Independence* report stated in 2005, these trends have "led to a fear that promising prospective scientists will choose not to pursue a career in academic biomedical research and, instead, opt for career paths that provide a greater chance for independence" (National Research Council, 2005, p. 1). The concern is perhaps even greater today, threatening an enterprise that in 2014 supported a total of 854,000 jobs across the country, accounted for more than $550 billion in direct economic output and nearly $660 billion in indirect economic output, and generated more than $67 billion in tax revenues for state and federal governments (TEConomy Partners, 2016).

The patchwork of measures to address the challenges facing young scientists that has emerged over the years has allowed the U.S. biomedical enterprise to continue to make significant scientific and medical advances. These measures, however, have not resolved the structural vulnerabilities in the system, and in some cases come at a great opportunity cost for young scientists. As a result, the career path to becoming an independent researcher is increasingly seen as perilous. These unresolved issues could diminish the nation's ability to recruit the best minds from all sectors of the U.S. population to careers in biomedical research and raise concerns about a system that may favor increasingly conservative research proposals over high-risk, innovative ideas.

The committee is not the first group to address these concerns and to suggest solutions in a report such as this. Before developing a new set of recommendations, the committee investigated the conclusions from these earlier reports (see Appendix B) to understand why the problems have not only persisted but also grown in intensity in the face of decades of thoughtful recommendations and growing stakeholder attention.

The committee identified several impediments to progress over the years, many of them likely working in concert. One impediment has been a constraint on resources. NIH funding has declined 22 percent in real dollars since 2003.[4] While other sources, including federal government agencies such as the National Science Foundation, U.S. Department of Agriculture, and Department of Defense, as well as external organizations such as philanthropic foundations, also provide support for biomedical researchers, NIH is the predominant funder. This reduction in available funds for research has constrained NIH's efforts to address the increasing barriers to biomedical research. Although Congress increased funding for NIH by $2 billion in each of fiscal years 2016 and 2017,[5] this only returned NIH funding to the level in real dollars that existed immediately prior

---

[4] See http://faseb.org/Science-Policy--Advocacy-and-Communications/Federal-Funding-Data/NIH-Research-Funding-Trends.aspx (accessed February 2, 2018).

[5] See http://faseb.org/Science-Policy--Advocacy-and-Communications/Federal-Funding-Data/NIH-Research-Funding-Trends.aspx (accessed February 2, 2018).

to sequestration, and the majority of the increases are dedicated to specific initiatives rather than NIH's broad research portfolio.

Second, there has been an absence of shared responsibility for the biomedical research system (Daniels, 2015). Many stakeholders tend to hold the federal government responsible for this system, placing blame for failures at the feet of NIH, the principal funder of biomedical research. Doing so, however, obscures the important role that other organizations, particularly universities, must play in developing and implementing solutions. The committee's review of the implementation of past recommendations revealed that NIH has been more responsive than other stakeholders—namely universities and research institutions—in adopting reforms. It has been too easy for stakeholders other than NIH to ignore or pay superficial attention to the recommendations repeatedly made in periodic reports. In addition, without a mechanism for shared oversight of the system, institutions acting unilaterally will fail to make progress to solve what are often shared systemic problems.

Third, a lack of comprehensive and easily available data about the biomedical research system itself has impaired progress on addressing these problems. The opacity of the system has prevented students and trainees from making informed decisions about their training and career options as well as hindered institutions' and policymakers' ability to decide with confidence how to proceed with policy and funding reforms to ensure the system's vibrancy and responsiveness.

Finally, the sands of the biomedical research enterprise are rapidly shifting. Since the release of earlier reports and their calls for reform, the funding landscape, demographic trends, and scientific priorities in science and industry have changed. The nature of research itself has evolved: team science, with its attendant premium on collaboration in multi-investigator and multidisciplinary projects, is ascendant; the growing use of pre-prints enables quick disclosure of research results; experimentation with hybrid business models blend traditional research institutes and for-profit companies; and the emergence of data sciences and online connectivity accelerates the pace at which experiments can be conducted.

The committee took its mandate seriously. Congress, NIH, scientific societies, and U.S. research institutions are acutely aware of the frailties of the current biomedical research environment and have put forth many recommendations, so there is a heightened sense of urgency to address the problems.

To meet its mandate, the committee developed recommendations that attend to the research ecosystem not only as it exists now, but also as it is likely to evolve during the next 10 years. This report discusses the current biomedical research ecosystem and its challenges, informed by new insights into the workforce from NIH and independent scholars, and proposes several substantive and structural reforms for stakeholders across the research enterprise. These reforms chart a path to a biomedical research enterprise that is competitive, rigorous, fair, and dynamic, and can attract the best minds from across the country. In such an enterprise

- All relevant institutions assume a role that reflects their interests and stake in the system, and mechanisms for shared oversight enable sustained and collaborative reform.
- Trainees and newly independent investigators receive accurate and timely information about their training and career prospects through mentorship and career counseling that aligns with their aspirations.
- Early-stage investigators are presented with stable and attractive career options, and robust roles exist for scientists inside and outside of the traditional academic faculty position.
- Policy experimentation and assessment are core concepts of the system, leading to the development and implementation of programs and policies that respond to investigators' needs at all stages of their careers.

To that end, the committee offers the following recommendations, grouped by report chapter:

Chapter 3: Transparency, Shared Responsibility, and Sustainability

Recommendation 3.1
Congress should establish a Biomedical Research Enterprise Council (BREC) to address ongoing challenges confronting the Next Generation of Biomedical Researchers. The BREC would exercise ongoing collective guardianship of the biomedical enterprise and function as a forum for sustained coordination, consultation, problem-solving, and assessment of progress toward implementation of the recommendations put forth in this report.

Recommendation 3.2
All stakeholders in the biomedical research enterprise—universities, research institutions, government laboratories, and biomedical industries—should promote, document, and disseminate their existing and planned efforts to reduce the barriers to recruiting and retaining diverse researchers at all stages of career development.

Recommendation 3.3
Biomedical research institutions should collect, analyze, and disseminate comprehensive data on outcomes, demographics, and career aspirations of biomedical pre- and postdoctoral researchers using common standards and definitions as developed by the institutions in concert with the National Institutes of Health (NIH). To incentivize compliance, NIH should make collection and publication of these data a requirement for additional NIH funding. This requirement should be phased-in over a 5-year period.

Recommendation 3.4
The National Science Foundation (NSF) should develop and implement a plan to improve sector-wide data collection and analysis in a manner that is easily accessible by policymakers and integrates data from numerous other sources. NSF should expeditiously link the Survey of Doctorate Recipients and the Survey of Earned Doctorates to U.S. Census data, and those linked data, under strict confidentiality protocols, should be made available for qualified researchers to use at Federal Statistical Research Data Centers to better understand the biomedical workforce.

Recommendation 3.5
Congress should consider increasing the National Institutes of Health (NIH) budget specifically to support implementation of the recommendations in this report and should provide sustained support for NIH's recently announced Next Generation Researchers Initiative.

Chapter 4: Transitioning to Independence

Recommendation 4.1
Research institutions, principal investigators (PIs), and federal funding agencies should each play their part to support transitions from Ph.D.'s, M.D.'s, and M.D.-Ph.D.'s to research independence by providing every postdoctoral researcher, regardless of the support mechanism or training location, with a high-quality training experience that prepares them for success in their chosen career. To achieve this overarching objective:

- The National Institutes of Health (NIH) should require the inclusion of an institutional training and mentoring plan as a component of the "Resources and Environment" reported on research and training grant applications. In addition, NIH should require PIs to provide a postdoctoral research training and mentoring plan in all grant proposals, as well as updates on those plans in annual and interim research performance progress reports for funded proposals.
- Research institutions should provide evidence to NIH of formal training of faculty mentors of postdoctoral trainees.
- Research institutions should introduce a mechanism to facilitate career guidance counseling for all postdoctoral researchers. This mechanism would preferably begin in the first year but must occur no later than the third year of postdoctoral training. Such guidance should assess the postdoctoral researchers' progress and evaluate alignment of their career aspirations with career prospects.
- NIH should increase the Ruth L. Kirschstein National Research Service Award (NRSA) starting salary for new postdoctoral researchers to $52,700 (in 2018 dollars), with annual adjustments for inflation and for

cost-of-living increases tied to the Personal Consumption Expenditure Index. Research institutions should adjust their base postdoctoral salary annually to match the corresponding NRSA rate, with adjustments based on local cost-of-living, and they should harmonize benefits for all postdoctoral scholars regardless of support mechanism.
- Research institutions should levy a fee of at least $1,000 per year, to be paid by the host investigator, for each postdoctoral fellow on all biomedical research grants. Funds from the fee would be used to support effective training and professional development programs for postdoctoral researchers, as well as effective training of mentors. Research institutions should report publicly on the use of the money generated by this fee.
- All research institutions should, following best practices, identify or provide an institutional ombudsperson to resolve fairly and expeditiously conflicts and concerns between PIs and postdoctoral researchers related to training experiences.

Recommendation 4.2
The National Institutes of Health (NIH) should expand existing awards or create new competitive awards to support postdoctoral researchers' advancement of their own independent research and to support professional development toward an independent research career. Both domestic and foreign postdoctoral researchers should be eligible for these awards. Over the next 5 years, NIH should incrementally and steadily increase by 5-fold the number of individual research fellowship awards (F-type) and career development (K-type) awards for postdoctoral researchers. The award recipients' home institutions should provide them with benefits commensurate to those provided to postdoctoral researchers supported on NIH research project grants and appropriate to their level of experience. The increase should not come at the expense of institutional training grants. The indirect cost recovery rate earned by K-type and training grant awards should be increased to 16 percent.

Recommendation 4.3
The National Institutes of Health (NIH) should phase in a cap (3 years suggested) on salary support for all postdoctoral researchers funded by NIH research project grants (RPGs) based on the following considerations:

- The cap should not apply to time spent on fellowships or career development awards;
- The phase-in should occur only after NIH undertakes a robust pilot study (or studies) of sufficient size and duration to assess the feasibility of this policy and provide opportunities to revise it;
- The pilot study (or studies) should be coupled to action on recommendation 4.2, which calls for an increase in individual F and K awards that are not restricted to U.S. citizens and permanent residents;

- The pilot study (or studies) should assess potential benefits as well as potential deleterious consequences of such a cap for postdoctoral researchers, with special emphasis on women, underrepresented racial and ethnic minorities, and individuals with disabilities; early-stage independent investigators; and research creativity;
- A short extension of RPG support can be requested, with sufficient justification, to offset time lost because of unplanned circumstances (e.g., illness, lab disaster) or parental responsibilities; and
- Postdoctoral researchers should be allowed sufficient time between their last fellowship decision and the termination of their funding on RPGs to enable smooth career transitions.

Recommendation 4.4
Postdoctoral training should be limited to 5 years, after which time any postdoctoral researcher continuing in the same laboratory should be shifted to employment as a staff scientist with increased salary and benefits as appropriate for a permanent staff member.

Recommendation 4.5
Congress and the National Institutes of Health (NIH) should create and expand existing entrepreneurial and private-sector opportunities to attract and support the next generation of biomedical and behavioral researchers.

- Congress should revise the Small Business Innovation Research (SBIR)/Small Business Technology Transfer (STTR) program to enable NIH to create a novel ecosystem that fosters entrepreneurship for next generation biomedical scientists, facilitates women- and minority-owned entrepreneurship, and supports fulfillment of NIH's mission across the private sector.
- Congress should extend/establish an employment tax credit to research and development (R&D) firms for hiring recently minted Ph.D.'s, M.D.'s, and M.D.-Ph.D.'s. and make the credit higher for small- to medium-sized R&D firms and firms that recruit into R&D activity for the first time.

Chapter 5: Building a Better Ecosystem for Independence

Recommendation 5.1
The National Institutes of Health (NIH) should invest in strengthening the research funding landscape for the next generation of investigators.

- To promote innovative research with high potential for groundbreaking discoveries, NIH should expand the number of NIH Director's New Innovator Awards (DP2) and similar programs funded by individual NIH Institutes and Centers.

- NIH should ensure that the duration of all R01 research grants supporting early-stage investigators (ESIs) is no less than 5 years to enable the establishment of resilient independent research programs. NIH Institutes and Centers should monitor the effect of this change on the availability of funds for other research project grants and should experiment with further extensions of the duration of R01 awards for ESIs.
- To avoid dis-incentivizing research collaboration, those ESIs who participate in multi-principal investigator (PI) submissions prior to receiving their own R01 grants should retain their ESI status unless serving as a co-PI on a funded multi-PI award provides them with R01-equivalent funds for their own research.
- NIH should expand the Pathways to Independence (K99/R00) award, with a priority on fostering independence through career development, including the development of an innovative and independent research project orginally conceived of and executed by the applicant, rather than additional or new training.

Recommendation 5.2
The National Institutes of Health (NIH) should continue to improve the peer review process to optimize the evaluation of applications submitted by early-stage and early experienced investigators in the Next Generation Researchers Initiative. This action would especially benefit investigators from underrepresented groups. NIH should revise the biosketch requirement to focus peer review on recent contributions and accomplishments and should continue to test effective practices to reduce the effects of implicit bias on the review process and to increase the diversity of reviewers.

Recommendation 5.3
Research institutions and the National Institutes of Health should develop mechanisms to increase the number of individuals in staff scientist positions to provide more stable, non-faculty research opportunities for the next generation of researchers. Research institutions should experiment with providing career tracks with clearly defined review and promotion processes, as well as opportunities for professional development. Individuals in a staff scientist track should receive a salary and benefits commensurate with their experience and responsibilities.

Recommendation 5.4
The National Institutes of Health (NIH), research institutions, and principal investigators should share responsibility for increasing the diversity of and promoting the inclusion of early-career researchers.

- To promote diversity and inclusion at the junior faculty level, NIH should require an institutional diversity and inclusion plan as a compo-

nent of the institutional resources reported on research grants supporting trainees.
- To promote diversity and inclusion of research trainees, principal investigators should provide a diversity and inclusion plan in their grant proposals and should provide updates in progress reports if funded.

Recommendation 5.5
The National Institutes of Health should allocate funds from its Next Generation Researchers Initiative to expand the number of Research Supplements to Promote Diversity in Health-Related Research (PA-16-288). These should be awarded to underrepresented minority (URM) early-stage investigators and URM investigators who have not been awarded a research project grant and seek to collaborate with funded investigators on new but related research projects. Proposals must clearly detail how the collaboration will result in a grant proposal by the URM investigator. To best support this career stage, awards should be enhanced with funds for supplies, equipment, professional development, and mentoring. The eligibility criteria for these diversity supplements should reflect only the URM populations specified by the National Science Foundation for the biomedical research enterprise.

Recommendation 5.6
The National Institutes of Health (NIH) should make the Loan Repayment Programs available to all individuals pursuing biomedical physician-scientist researcher careers, regardless of their research area or clinical specialty. NIH should increase the monetary value of loan repayment to reflect the debt burden of current medical trainees. NIH should also continue implementation of the recommendations laid out in the 2014 *NIH Physician-Scientist Workforce Working Group Report*. NIH should test new strategies and expand effective approaches to increase the pool of early-stage physician-scientists.

Chapter 6: Experimentation and Innovation

Recommendation 6.1
Congress and the National Institutes of Health should promote innovative pilot projects on the part of research institutions and other stakeholders that seek to improve and accelerate transitions into independent careers. A Next Generation Researcher Innovation Fund should be created to support these experimental projects.

Recommendation 6.2
The National Institutes of Health should enhance the use of its Institutes and Centers as vehicles to pilot new mechanisms designed to support the independence of early-career researchers and thereby strengthen its capacity for innovation more

broadly. The Biomedical Research Enterprise Council proposed in recommendation 3.1 should monitor and evaluate those efforts.

Many of these recommendations will require new policies or funding mechanisms, and others encompass structural norms that reflect an effort to shift to a new paradigm, one premised on multi-stakeholder involvement, transparency, multiple pathways for research success, and a tradition of evidence-based experimentation and innovation. In this manner, the committee seeks to offer recommendations for reform and for the conditions necessary for their adoption, assessment, and ongoing adaptation and responsiveness, with the goal of creating a biomedical research enterprise that is truly equipped to promote the independence, creativity, and innovation of our scientists, for the benefit not only of the next generation of researchers and the generations to follow, but also the health and economic strength of the nation.

REFERENCES

Cyranoski, D., N. Gilbert, H. Ledford, A. Nayar, and M. Yahia. 2011. Education: The PhD factory. *Nature* 472(7343):276-279.

Daniels, R. 2015. A generation at risk: Young investigators and the future of the biomedical workforce. *Proceedings of the National Academy of Sciences of the United States of America* 112(2): 313-318.

Edwards, M. A., and S. Roy. 2017. Academic research in the 21st century: Maintaining scientific integrity in a climate of perverse incentives and hypercompetition. *Environmental Engineering Science* 34(1):51-61.

National Research Council. 2005. *Bridges to independence: Fostering the independence of new investigators in biomedical research*. Washington, DC: The National Academies Press.

National Science Board. 2018. *Science and engineering indicators, 2018*. Alexandria, VA: National Science Foundation.

TEConomy Partners. 2016. *The economic impact of the U.S. biopharmaceutical industry*. Washington, DC: Pharmaceutical Research and Manufacturers of America.

1

Introduction and Overview

Thirteen years ago, the National Academies sponsored a report called *Bridges to Independence: Fostering the Independence of New Investigators in Biomedical Research* (National Research Council, 2005). Highlighting data showing that the age at which science investigators receive their first research grant was increasing, and that the number and percentage of grants awarded to young researchers was decreasing, the report voiced concern about the vitality of the U.S. biomedical[1] research enterprise and, in particular, the fate of early-career investigators. The report explained the following:

> Academic biomedical researchers are therefore spending long periods of time at the beginning of their careers unable to set their own research directions or establish their independence. This has led to a fear that promising prospective scientists will choose not to pursue a career in academic biomedical research and, instead, opt for career paths that provide a greater chance for independence. This "crisis of expectation" has severe and troubling implications for the future of biomedical research in the United States. (National Research Council, 2005, p. 1)

These concerns have not lessened in the years since the *Bridges to Independence* study. Congress included language in the 2016 Consolidated Appropriations Act[2] requiring the director of the National Institutes of Health (NIH) to enter into an agreement with the National Academies to produce

---

[1] In this report, "biomedical" refers to the full range of biological, biomedical, behavioral, and health sciences supported by the National Institutes of Health.

[2] Consolidated Appropriations Act, 2016, P.L. 114-113, 129 Stat. 2608 (2015). Available at https://www.congress.gov/bill/114th-congress/house-bill/2029/text (accessed January 19, 2018).

(A) an evaluation of the legislative, administrative, educational, and cultural barriers faced by the next generation of researchers; (B) an evaluation of the impact of federal budget constraints on the next generation of researchers; and (C) recommendations for the implementation of policies to incentivize, improve entry into, and sustain careers in research for the next generation of researchers, including proposed policies for agencies and academic institutions.

In addition, Congress included in the 21st Century Cures Act of 2016[3] a section titled "Investing in the Next Generation of Researchers" that requires the NIH director to "[p]romote policies and programs within the National Institutes of Health that are focused on improving opportunities for new researchers and promoting earlier research independence, including existing policies and programs, as appropriate" and to "develop, modify, or prioritize policies, as needed, within the National Institutes of Health to promote opportunities for new researchers and earlier research independence, such as policies to increase opportunities for new researchers to receive funding, enhance training and mentorship programs for researchers, and enhance workforce diversity." The bill also called for the NIH director to "take into consideration the recommendations made by the National Academies of Sciences, Engineering, and Medicine as part of the comprehensive study on policies affecting the next generation of researchers."

As a result of that directive, the Board on Higher Education and Workforce (BHEW) of the National Academies of Sciences, Engineering, and Medicine convened an ad hoc committee tasked with evaluating factors that influence transitions into independent research careers in the biomedical and behavioral sciences, and developing recommendations to improve those transitions (see Box 1-1).

WORK OF THE COMMITTEE

Throughout the 18-month study, the committee held five meetings, including three held outside Washington, DC, in Cambridge, MA, San Francisco, CA, and Baltimore, MD, to allow for a diversity of input from university researchers and other stakeholders (see Appendix E for the meeting agendas). In addition to issues identified during the public sessions, the committee considered a wide range of articles in the published literature and a select number of reports issued over the past 20 years that have focused on the biomedical and behavioral sciences research workforces, postdoctoral researchers, and young investigators in the early stages of their careers (see Appendix B for a list of those reports).

The committee was acutely aware that it was not the first to review the state of early-career investigators in the biomedical workforce and that it was writing against the backdrop of a series of prior reports. Early in its deliberations, the committee compiled a list of recommendations included in major reports issued

---

[3] 21st Century Cures Act, P.L. 114-225 § 2021, 130 Stat. 1051, 1052 (2016). Available at https://www.gpo.gov/fdsys/pkg/PLAW-114publ255/content-detail.html (accessed January 19, 2018).

> **BOX 1-1**
> **Statement of Task**
>
> An ad hoc committee, overseen by the Board on Higher Education and Workforce (BHEW), will examine the policy and programmatic steps that the nation can undertake to ensure the successful launch and sustainment of careers among the next generation of researchers in the biomedical and behavioral sciences, including the full range of health sciences supported by the NIH. The committee will examine evidence-based programs and policies that can reduce barriers to, and create more opportunities, incentives, and pathways for successful transitions to independent research careers. It will also examine factors that influence the stability and sustainability of the early stages of independent research careers. The study will include:
>
> 1. An evaluation of the barriers that prospective researchers encounter as they transition to independent research careers. Such barriers may include inadequate career guidance and support, insufficient access to fellowships and traineeships that would provide broad exposure to research experiences, inability to compete successfully for initial research grant awards, and postdoctoral experiences that limit options for pursuing independent research careers;
> 2. An evaluation of the impact of federal policies and budgets, including federal agency policies and procedures regarding research grant awards, on opportunities for prospective researchers to successfully transition into independent research careers and to secure their all-important first and second major research grants; and
> 3. An evaluation of the extent to which employers (industry, government agencies and labs, academic institutions, and others) can facilitate smooth transitions for early career investigators into independent research careers.
>
> The committee will issue a report summarizing the results of these evaluations with federal and institutional policy recommendations to improve the transition to independent careers for the next generation of researchers in the biomedical and behavioral sciences.

by the National Academies, NIH, and the Federation of American Societies of Experimental Biology (FASEB), and it assembled information on the actions or inactions of stakeholders in response to the recommendations. The responses to prior recommendations are discussed throughout the report and are listed in Appendix B. The committee also received input from NIH on past and current initiatives focused on early-stage investigators.

The committee also collected data about the biomedical workforce from a range of sources. Most prominently, the committee made numerous requests for data from NIH, which responded in a diligent and timely manner. The data provided important insights that guided deliberations and informed the process for developing recommendations and identifying the multiple stakeholders linked to the recommendations. Much of these data are discussed in Chapter 2.

Furthermore, recognizing that the rest of the world is not sitting still, and to gain perspective on the issues facing other biomedical research systems around the world and their approaches in addressing concerns about their early independent investigators, the committee commissioned expert reports on policies under way to improve the next generation of research in five other regions: Canada, China, the European Union, the United Kingdom, and Singapore. The authors of these reports presented their findings to the committee, and their analyses informed deliberations.[4]

As an additional means to gather input, the committee released a "Dear Colleague" letter, inviting the biomedical research community at large to provide input on recommendations proposed in the published literature (see Appendix C). BHEW staff established a website, http://www.nas.edu/nextgeninput, where the community could provide input. The committee received feedback from a range of individuals and professional organizations that further informed its deliberations.[5]

SCOPE OF THE STUDY

Consistent with its Statement of Task, the committee focused its efforts on the specific challenges facing the next generation of investigators as they transition from training to independent research careers. This transition period does not exist in isolation from the remainder of the biomedical research career path. To complete its task, the committee looked beyond this transition period to other career stages that are relevant to the question at hand—for example, what information will allow trainees to successfully transition to independence, or the implications of reforms for mid-career investigators.

In defining "independent research careers," the committee was guided by the 2005 National Academies report, *Bridges to Independence* (National Research Council, 2005, p. 3), which defined an "independent investigator" as someone who

> . . . enjoys independence of thought—the freedom to define the problem of interest and/or to choose or develop the best strategies and approaches to address that problem. Under this definition, an independent scientist may work alone, as the intellectual leader of a research group, or as a member of a consortium of investigators each contributing distinct expertise. Specifically, we do not intend "independence" to mean necessarily "isolated" or "solitary," or to imply "self-sustaining" or "separately funded."

---

[4] These reports are available on the study website http://www.nas.edu/NextGen (accessed March 15, 2018).

[5] The compiled, anonymized responses are available on the study website http://www.nas.edu/NextGen (accessed March 15, 2018).

Regarding the transition to independence of biomedical scientists, the committee deliberately considered academic faculty positions at research universities and the multiplicity of positions in government and industry where scientists currently conduct their research. Indeed, the committee believes that the narrow focus in the system on academic careers is one source of the problems affecting the next generation of scientists.

For ease of narrative, the committee refers to the biomedical sciences or biomedical research through this report; however, this report extends as well to the full range of health sciences supported by NIH. Although most of the training and NIH-funded research in the biomedical sciences is conducted at research universities, the recommendations put forth in this report, except where specified, extend to the broader spectrum of research institutions outside of academia or private industry where the next generation of biomedical researchers is trained and where research is conducted.

STRUCTURE OF THE REPORT

The remainder of this report addresses the committee's activities, findings, and recommendations. Chapter 2 describes the challenges facing young investigators at each stage of their developing careers and why it is important to address those challenges. The four chapters that follow arrange the recommendations by theme: Chapter 3 on Transparency, Shared Responsibility, and Sustainability; Chapter 4 on Transitions to Independence; Chapter 5 on Building a Better Ecosystem for Independence; and Chapter 6 on Innovation and Experimentation. The committee then offers some concluding thoughts in Chapter 7.

REFERENCE

National Research Council. 2005. *Bridges to independence: Fostering the independence of new investigators in biomedical research*. Washington, DC: The National Academies Press.

2

The Landscape for the Next Generation of Researchers

The career trajectory of an independent researcher in the biomedical[1] or behavioral sciences has undergone striking changes in recent decades, as have the training, research, and funding environments they inhabit. These changes affect the foundation of the biomedical research enterprise, specifically the researchers who discover new knowledge, drive innovation, and promote worldwide health.

In this chapter, the committee describes the promise, opportunities, and challenges of the current landscape for the next generation of researchers as they pursue a path to independence. The discussion is divided into the several phases of that path—commencing with doctoral and medical training; the move for many to postdoctoral experiences; the transition to independent research opportunities in academic and non-academic domains; and the pursuit of funding and other challenges that investigators face as they seek to establish a sustainable and fruitful career.

DOCTORAL AND MEDICAL TRAINING IN BIOMEDICAL RESEARCH

As of fall 2015, more than 140,000 students were enrolled in U.S. graduate school programs in the biomedical and health sciences.[2] Of that population,

---

[1] In this report, "biomedical" refers to the full range of biological, biomedical, behavioral, and health sciences supported by the National Institutes of Health (NIH).

[2] National Science Foundation (NSF). Survey of Graduate Students and Postdoctorates in Science and Engineering, Table 9: Graduate students in science, engineering, and health in all institutions, by detailed field: 2010–15. https://ncsesdata.nsf.gov/datatables/gradpostdoc/2015/html/GSS2015_DST_09.html (accessed December 14, 2017). Included in this accounting are the following fields:

19

64 percent were women, 20 percent held temporary visas, and 19 percent were from racial and ethnic groups traditionally underrepresented in science and engineering.[3] In the same year, more than 11,000 biological, biomedical, and health students earned their Ph.D. or equivalent doctorate degree.[4] Of those doctorate recipients, 56 percent were women, 24 percent held temporary visas, and 9 percent were from traditionally underrepresented minority groups. In 2016, approximately 19,000 people in the United States received a medical degree, with 46 percent women and 10 percent from underrepresented minority groups.[5] Of those who graduated with a medical degree in the United States in 2016, 602 graduated with an M.D.-Ph.D., and, of those, 38 percent were female[6] and 5 percent were from underrepresented minority groups.[7]

The nature of doctoral training in the United States is outside the scope of this report, but is the topic of another National Academies study.[8] However, a few observations about doctoral training periods are relevant to the mandate of this committee. First, the median time from matriculation to a Ph.D. in the life sciences was 6.7 years in 2015, declining from 7.7 years in 1990.[9] Although the age at which researchers secure their first major NIH grant has increased during the past several decades, this increase is not due to a longer duration of doctoral training. However, the average length of training for M.D.-Ph.D. recipients has increased, from 6.6 years in the 1980s to 8 years in 2012 (National Institutes of Health, 2014), so increases in the average age of research independence for M.D.-Ph.D. recipients could be connected to longer training periods.

---

anatomy, biochemistry, biology, biometry and epidemiology, biophysics, cell and molecular biology, entomology and parasitology, genetics, microbiology, immunology, virology, nutrition, pathology, pharmacology and toxicology, physiology, biosciences, neurobiology and neuroscience, and health.

[3] NSF defines underrepresented minorities as comprising three racial or ethnic minority groups (blacks, Hispanics, and American Indians or Alaska Natives) whose representation in science and engineering education or employment is smaller than their representation in the U.S. population. NSF. Women, Minorities, and Persons with Disabilities in Science and Engineering 2017. https://www.nsf.gov/statistics/2017/nsf17310/digest/glossary-and-key-to-acronyms/ (accessed February 7, 2018).

[4] NSF. Survey of Earned Doctorates 2015, Table 12: Doctorate recipients, by subfield of study: 2005-2015. https://www.nsf.gov/statistics/2017/nsf17306/datatables/tab-12.htm (accessed December 14, 2017).

[5] American Association of Medical Colleges (AAMC). Table B-4: Total U.S. medical school graduates by race/ethnicity and sex, 2012-2013 through 2016-2017. https://www.aamc.org/download/321536/data/factstableb4.pdf (accessed January 24, 2018).

[6] Data provided courtesy of AAMC and available from public access file.

[7] AAMC. Table B-13: Race/ethnicity responses (alone and in combination) of MD-PhD graduates of U.S. medical schools, 2012-2013 through 2016-2017. https://www.aamc.org/download/450638/data/factstableb13.pdf (accessed January 24, 2018).

[8] National Academies of Sciences, Engineering, and Medicine. Graduate Education for the 21st Century. http://www.nas.edu/GradEd (accessed February 7, 2018).

[9] NSF. Survey of Earned Doctorates 2015, Table 31: Median years to doctorate, by broad field of study: Selected years, 1990–2015. https://www.nsf.gov/statistics/2017/nsf17306/datatables/tab-31.htm (accessed December 14, 2017).

Second, the number of individuals obtaining Ph.D.'s in the biomedical sciences has steadily increased, and the majority of them will continue their training after receiving their degrees. A recent analysis showed that the annual number of individuals receiving a biomedical Ph.D. more than doubled during the period 1980 to 2010, while the percentage of individuals starting their careers in a postdoctoral position largely remained steady at about 82.5 percent (Kahn and Ginther, 2017). The increase in the number of Ph.D.'s, combined with the continued trend of biomedical doctorate recipients pursuing a postdoctoral experience after graduation, has contributed to a dramatic rise in the number of individuals in the United States in postdoctoral research positions.

THE POSTDOCTORAL RESEARCH EXPERIENCE

The postdoctoral experience is a temporary period of training following the award of a doctoral or medical degree to gain additional scientific, technical, and professional skills that advance the careers of Ph.D.'s, M.D.'s, and M.D.-Ph.D.'s. As discussed in the 2014 National Academies of Sciences report, *The Postdoctoral Experience Revisited*, the National Science Foundation (NSF), National Institutes of Health (NIH), Association of American Medical Colleges (AAMC), and the National Postdoctoral Association (NPA) all formalized definitions of postdoctoral researchers in the mid-2000s (National Academy of Sciences et al., 2014a). Their definitions and characterizations (updated for 2018) are provided in Box 2-1.

While receiving valuable research training, postdoctoral researchers play an indispensable role in the research enterprise, "performing a substantial portion of the nation's research in every setting" (Institute of Medicine et al., 2000, p. 10). Understanding their experiences and outcomes is challenging, however, because of well-documented problems with the available data (National Institutes of Health, 2012a, p. 9; National Academy of Sciences et al., 2014a). These challenges include inconsistent titles and definitions for postdoctoral researchers, as well as inconsistent data on their employment experiences, pay, benefits, and duration of their appointment across institutions. As a result, estimates of the total number of biomedical postdoctoral researchers in the United States range widely from 30,000 to 80,000. Some data sets, such as the NSF Survey of Graduate Students and Postdoctorates in Science and Engineering (GSS), count only postdoctoral researchers employed at U.S. degree-granting institutions and not those employed by industry or research institutions. There have been repeated calls to collect and disseminate demographic and outcomes data on postdoctoral populations to guide both individual and policy decisions, but no national efforts have been sustained. More recently, NSF has developed and piloted the Early Career Doctorates Survey to gather in-depth information about individuals who earned an initial doctoral degree within the past 10 years, including non-citizens as well as U.S. citizens and permanent residents.

> **BOX 2-1**
> **Postdoctoral Researcher: 2018 Definitions and Characterizations**
>
> - **National Science Foundation:** An individual who received a Ph.D., M.D., D.Sc. or equivalent degree less than five years ago, who is not a member of the faculty at the performing institution, and who is not reported under Senior Personnel above.
> - **National Institutes of Health:** An individual with a doctoral degree (PhD, MD, DDS, or the equivalent) who is engaged in a temporary period of mentored research and/or scholarly training for the purpose of acquiring the professional skills needed to pursue a career path of his or her choosing.
> - **Association of American Medical Colleges:** Postdoctoral training is an integral component of the preparation of scientists for career advancement as scientific professionals. Postdoctoral appointees typically join an institution to further their training in a chosen discipline after recently obtaining their terminal degree (e.g., Ph.D., M.D., D.V.M.). This training is conducted in an apprenticeship mode where she/he works under the supervision of an investigator who is qualified to fulfill the responsibilities of a mentor. The postdoctoral appointee may undertake scholarship, research, service, and teaching activities that together provide a training experience essential for career advancement.
> - **National Postdoctoral Association:** An individual holding a doctoral degree who is engaged in a temporary period of mentored research and/or scholarly training for the purpose of acquiring the professional skills needed to pursue a career path of his or her choosing.
>
> ---
>
> SOURCES:
> NSF: NSF 04-23 September 2004. Appendix F—Definitions of Categories of Personnel. https://www.nsf.gov/pubs/gpg/nsf04_23/appf.jsp (accessed February 7, 2018).
> NIH: NIH Office of Intramural Training and Education. Postdoc FAQs. https://www.training.nih.gov/resources/faqs/postdoc_irp (accessed February 7, 2018).
> AAMC: Compact Between Postdoctoral Appointees and Their Mentors. https://www.aamc.org/download/49852/data/postdoccompact.pdf (accessed February 7, 2018).
> NPA: What is a Postdoc? http://www.nationalpostdoc.org/?page=What_is_a_postdoc (accessed February 7, 2018).

Despite these data limitations, one can tease out some broad trends about the postdoctoral population at U.S. degree-granting institutions. The NSF GSS reported that nearly 39,000 individuals were working in postdoctoral positions in the biomedical and health sciences in 2015,[10] and the gender, race, and ethnicity

---

[10] NSF. Survey of Graduate Students and Postdoctorates in Science and Engineering, Table 43: Female postdoctoral appointees in science, engineering, and health in all institutions, by detailed field, citizenship, ethnicity, and race: 2015. https://ncsesdata.nsf.gov/datatables/gradpostdoc/2015/html/GSS2015_DST_43.html (accessed January 23, 2018). Included in this accounting are the following fields: anatomy, biochemistry, biology, biometry and epidemiology, biophysics, cell and molecular

of those postdoctoral researchers did not reflect the demographics of newly minted biomedical doctorates from that same year. While 56 percent of doctorate recipients in 2015 were women, only 46 percent of postdoctoral researchers in the same fields were women. In addition, 9 percent of the biomedical Ph.D.'s were awarded to individuals from underrepresented minority groups in 2015, but only 5 percent of postdoctoral researchers in those fields were from those same groups.

A substantial proportion of biomedical postdoctoral researchers are not U.S. citizens or permanent residents. Of the biomedical postdoctoral researchers included in the 2015 NSF GSS, 53 percent held temporary visas and 31 percent reported earning their degrees in a foreign country. Moreover, the origin of the degree was unknown for 33 percent of biomedical postdoctoral researchers surveyed the same year.[11] These percentages reflect both the openness of U.S. biomedical training and labor markets and the attractiveness of U.S. research careers to international scholars. It is also the case that some countries encourage recent Ph.D.'s to seek postdoctoral training in the United States.[12]

In the extramurally funded biomedical sciences, postdoctoral researchers at U.S. degree-granting institutions are supported largely by NIH funding mechanisms. In 2016, approximately 10 percent of postdoctoral researchers in the biomedical, behavioral, social, and clinical sciences were supported on federal fellowships and traineeships, such as the Ruth L. Kirschstein Individual National Research Service Award (NRSA) postdoctoral fellowship (F32), which provides support to individual postdoctoral fellows, and the Ruth L. Kirschstein Institutional NRSA training grant (T32), which provides support to institutions to develop training opportunities for selected individuals.[13] That same year, 46 percent of postdoctoral researchers were supported on a federal research grant, which is awarded to a principal investigator (PI) and supports individuals selected by the PI, and 44 percent received non-federal support. Of postdoctoral researchers specifically supported by NIH in 2016, approximately 79 percent of them were supported on research project grants (RPGs) and 19 percent were supported on a fellowship or traineeship.[14]

---

biology, entomology and parasitology, genetics, microbiology, immunology, virology, nutrition, pathology, pharmacology and toxicology, physiology, biosciences, neurobiology and neuroscience, and health.

[11] NSF. Survey of Graduate Students and Postdoctorates in Science and Engineering 2015, Table 48: Postdoctoral appointees in science, engineering, and health in all institutions, by detailed field and origin of doctoral degree: 2015. https://ncsesdata.nsf.gov/gradpostdoc/2015/html/GSS2015_DST_48.html (accessed February 7, 2018).

[12] See the international commissioned papers for this study, available at http://www.nas.edu/NextGen/resources.

[13] NIH Data Book. Primary Source of Support for Postdoctorates. https://report.nih.gov/NIH-Databook/Charts/Default.aspx?showm=YandchartId=263andcatId=20 (accessed December 14, 2017).

[14] NSF. Survey of Graduate Students and Postdoctorates in Science and Engineering 2016, Table 41: Postdoctoral appointees in science, engineering, and health in all institutions, by field, primary source of support, and primary mechanism of support: 2016. https://ncsesdata.nsf.gov/gradpostdoc/2016/html/GSS2016_DST_41.html (accessed March 6, 2018).

NIH training grants, such as individual F32 and institutional T32 awards, are restricted to U.S. citizens and permanent residents, undergo peer review of the research and training plan, and include stipulations for professional development and mentoring by eligible mentors. For postdoctoral researchers, obtaining a fellowship is often considered a step toward professional independence, but significantly fewer postdoctoral researchers are supported on fellowships and training grants than on RPGs. In fact, the number of postdoctoral researchers supported on F32 grants was lower in 2016 (516 awards) than any year since 1998.[15] For postdoctoral researchers supported on an RPG, NIH states, "Staff in postdoctoral positions engaged in research, while not generally pursuing an additional degree, are expected to be actively engaged in their training and career development under their research appointments as Post-Docs."[16] However, there is neither a requirement to include a plan for training and professional development in the grant application, an assessment of the PI as a mentor, nor any other formal mechanism to ensure quality training and mentorship opportunities. In 2014 NIH implemented a policy that RPG Research Performance Progress Reports (RPPRs) must include a brief description of how and whether Individual Development Plans (IDPs) are used to manage the career development of students and postdoctoral researchers associated with that award.[17] These deficiencies contribute to a longstanding concern about a disparity in the treatment of postdoctoral researchers between RPGs and training grants (National Research Council, 2005). Moreover, because only U.S. citizens or nationals or lawful permanent residents are eligible for NIH-funded fellowships or training grants, postdoctoral researchers from other countries are significantly less likely to receive mandated training and professional development.

The fastest growing and second most prevalent source of postdoctoral support at degree-granting institutions is non-federal organizations, such as philanthropies, research centers, universities, the private sector, and professional societies.[18] The Health Research Alliance, a national consortium of more than 70 nongovernmental, nonprofit funders of biomedical research and training, provided $866 million in research awards in 2012.[19] Of that amount, 44 percent was for early-career development and training, including programs such as the American Cancer Society's Postdoctoral Fellowship Award and the Damon Runyon Cancer Research Foundation's Postdoctoral Research Fellowship. These organizations try to identify gaps in

---

[15] NIH Data Book. Kirschstein-NRSA post-doctoral fellowships (F32): Competing applications, awards, and success rates. https://report.nih.gov/NIHDatabook/Charts/Default.aspx?showm=YandchartId=106andcatId=13 (accessed February 9, 2018).

[16] NIH. OMB Clarifies Guidance on the Dual Role of Student and Postdoctoral Researchers. https://grants.nih.gov/grants/guide/notice-files/NOT-OD-15-008.html (accessed February 7, 2018).

[17] See https://grants.nih.gov/grants/guide/notice-files/not-od-14-113.html (accessed March 16, 2018).

[18] NIH Data Book. Primary Source of Support for Postdoctorates. https://report.nih.gov/NIH-Databook/Charts/Default.aspx?showm=YandchartId=263andcatId=20 (accessed December 14, 2017).

[19] See https://issuu.com/kfowlerdesign/docs/hra_report_grantsanalysis_highres (accessed January 19, 2018).

funding where they can provide "risk capital" for innovative but risky initiatives, an agenda that includes supporting unproven but promising postdoctoral researchers and other early-career researchers who, "because of their career stage and lack of track record, are unlikely to procure significant federal funding for their ideas until they are at a much later career stage."[20]

In addition to those postdoctoral researchers described above who work in degree-granting institutions, there are many employed in industry, national laboratories, and non-academic research institutions. The size of the postdoctoral workforce in those sectors is not clear, but the roles and experiences of these postdoctoral researchers and their peers in academia are notably different. According to the National Academies report *The Postdoctoral Experience Revisited* (National Academy of Sciences et al., 2014a, p.3), their "roles are better defined, salaries are higher, terms are shorter, and the connection to career development is clearer."

It is difficult to determine with accuracy the length of time researchers spend in their postdoctoral positions and whether that duration has changed over time. One recent analysis, however, found that the duration has held relatively constant over the past several decades at 4.5 years (Kahn and Ginther, 2017). There appeared to be a slight decrease in the duration after the late 1990s, perhaps attributable to a gradual move by some universities to cap postdoctoral periods at their institutions. Even so, approximately 20 percent of postdoctoral fellows in 2005 had spent 7 or more years in postdoctoral research positions (Kahn and Ginther, 2017). It is unclear whether these postdoctoral researchers had prolonged postdoctoral experiences because (1) they came from institutions with shorter doctoral training periods, (2) they required additional training because of their specific research areas, (3) they were in a "holding pattern" because of the scarce availability of independent academic research positions, or (4) other unknown reasons. Importantly, the data from this analysis are only included up to 2006, so it is unclear whether these trends persisted over the following decade. Despite calls in prior reports for improved data collection on postdoctoral researchers, it remains challenging to find comprehensive quantitative and qualitative data about the postdoctoral research experience.

Several surveys in recent years have revealed qualitative aspects of the postdoctoral experience. Respondents in a national survey of 1,002 American biological and life science postdoctoral researchers reported lower clarity on career goals during the postdoctoral experience than upon entry into or departure from Ph.D. programs (Gibbs et al., 2015). In a separate study, only 4 percent of biological and life sciences postdoctoral researchers reported feeling a "severe lack of information" regarding research careers in academia, but that number increased to 21 percent in government, 34 percent in established companies, and 42 percent in start-ups (Sauermann and Roach, 2016). Finally, those doctorates

---

[20] See https://www.healthra.org/download-resource/?resource-url=/wp-content/uploads/2013/08/Robertson_ebook.pdf (accessed March 16, 2018).

who had not thought about their careers at all were more likely to pursue a postdoctoral experience than those who had (Sauermann and Roach, 2016). These results are broadly consistent with prior reports that highlight a persistent lack of communication about the broad range of career prospects and educational and training opportunities for doctoral and postdoctoral researchers (National Academy of Sciences et al., 2014a).

NIH has developed initiatives to address the need for postdoctoral career development. For postdoctoral researchers supported on NRSA awards, NIH requires institutions to offer preparation for research-related and research-intensive careers in various sectors, such as academic institutions, government agencies, for-profit businesses, and private foundations.[21] In 2013, NIH launched the Strengthening the Biomedical Research Workforce program through the NIH Common Fund as one component of a trans-NIH strategy to enhance training opportunities for early-career scientists to prepare them for a variety of research-related career options.[22] A core component of this program is the NIH Director's Biomedical Research Workforce Innovation Awards to enhance biomedical research training, more commonly called the Broadening Experiences in Scientific Training (BEST) awards.[23] These 5-year awards are intended to support innovation in both graduate student and postdoctoral researcher training. Although a broad evaluation of BEST is not yet available, the awarded institutions convene annually to share data, develop best practices, and discuss program sustainability.

It is promising that multiple initiatives are aimed at providing postdoctoral researchers with career development opportunities, but an economic analysis of career paths for biomedical doctorates reveals that the postdoctoral experience can come at a substantial opportunity cost. Recent data indicate that postdoctoral training may not provide a positive financial return for more than a decade if the postdoctoral researcher later pursues jobs outside of academia. Biomedical Ph.D.'s in postdoctoral research positions earn an average of $45,000 per year for several years. In comparison, biomedical Ph.D.'s who enter the workforce immediately after degree attainment earn a median starting salary of $73,662. It can take 12 to 15 years after degree attainment for the postdoctoral research cohort to make up the lost earnings. The salary advantage in private industry for foregoing a postdoctoral position is especially pronounced for Ph.D.'s conducting biomedical research (Kahn and Ginther, 2017). Despite repeated recommendations to increase postdoctoral stipends and salaries (American Academy of Arts and Sciences, 2014; FASEB, 2015; McDowell et al., 2014; National Academy of Sciences et al., 2014a; National Institutes of Health, 2012a; National Research Council, 2011), the 2017 starting postdoctoral stipend of $47,484 for NRSA

---

[21] See https://grants.nih.gov/grants/guide/pa-files/PA-18-403.html (accessed December 14, 2017).

[22] See https://commonfund.nih.gov/workforce (accessed December 14, 2017).

[23] See https://grants.nih.gov/grants/guide/rfa-files/RFA-RM-12-022.html (accessed December 14, 2017).

grants remains below the National Academies 2014 recommended salary of $50,000 in 2014 dollars, or approximately $52,700 in 2018 dollars.[24]

Postdoctoral researchers in the United States face persistent and troubling challenges. First, they face fierce competition for a limited number of academic faculty positions. Second, they are a vulnerable part of the biomedical workforce because these positions are short-term and thus susceptible to fluctuations in federal research budgets. Third, although they seek these positions to enhance their skills, they are principally supported on RPGs in individual laboratories across the institution, which does not ensure quality mentoring and training experiences. At the core of concerns about the postdoctoral research experience is whether it provides value to postdoctoral researchers and prepares them for a variety of research careers outside of academia, and whether it proportionately and adequately supports diverse populations. Without comprehensive and longitudinal data on the postdoctoral population, however, it is difficult to develop evidence-based recommendations for improving the quality of the postdoctoral experience and recruiting an appropriate number of promising scientists from diverse populations into the biomedical research enterprise.

TRANSITION TO INDEPENDENT RESEARCH POSITIONS

In general, postdoctoral experience is considered necessary preparation for research positions in academia, but it does not guarantee advancement to such a position. According to one survey, 60 percent of postdoctoral researchers in biological and life sciences who graduated before 2013 reported that they accepted their position primarily to secure a faculty tenure-track position (Sauermann and Roach, 2016). However, another recent analysis showed that only 27.4 percent of employed individuals, regardless of their cohort, previously employed in biomedical postdoctoral research had tenure-track or tenured positions (Kahn and Ginther, 2017). The same mismatch between career aspiration and reality plays out more notably for recently trained cohorts, as studies show that greater than 50 percent of Ph.D.'s in the biological and life sciences rank a faculty research position as their desired career (Sauermann and Roach, 2012). As of 2013, however, only 18 percent of all U.S.-trained Ph.D.'s were employed in tenure-track or tenured positions 6 to 10 years after completing their Ph.D. training (Figure 2-1).

The percentage of Ph.D.'s in tenure-track positions has declined significantly in recent years. Partially contributing to this decline is increased hiring of new faculty in nontenure-eligible appointments.[25] According to Figure 2-1, in 1993, slightly greater than 10 percent of individuals were in tenure-track or tenured faculty positions within 5 years of degree attainment, but that percentage dropped to 6 percent by 2013. Only 18 percent of biomedical Ph.D.'s 6 to 10 years post

---

[24] See https://grants.nih.gov/grants/guide/notice-files/NOT-OD-16-131.html (accessed January 19, 2018).

[25] See https://www.aamc.org/download/434462/data/june2015aib.pdf (accessed December 14, 2017).

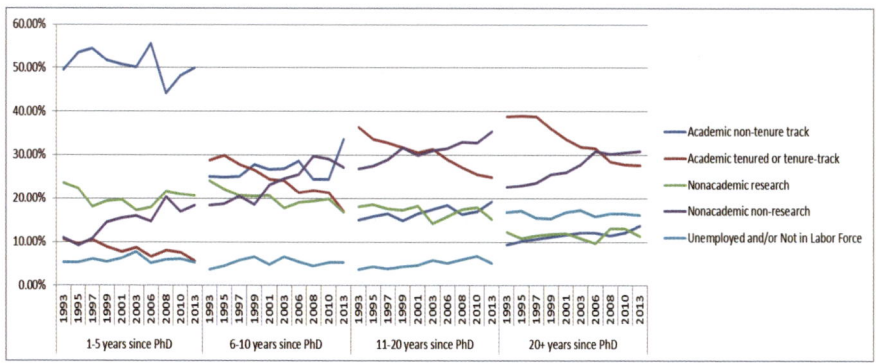

FIGURE 2-1 Percentage of U.S. trained biomedical individuals living in the United States, sector of employment by cohort and position, 1993-2013.
SOURCE: Prepared by Donna Ginther, University of Kansas (previously unpublished). The use of NSF data does not imply NSF endorsement of the research, research methods, or conclusions contained in this report.

degree attainment held academic tenure-track or tenured positions in 2013, compared to 29 percent in 1993.[26] An analysis from the AAMC supports a similar trend at medical colleges, where 73 percent of full-time basic science Ph.D. faculty were on tenure-eligible tracks in 2014, compared to 82 percent in 1984.[27]

As the percentage of biomedical Ph.D.'s in tenure-track or tenured faculty positions has declined, their representation has notably increased in two other sectors: academic non-tenure track positions and non-academic non-research positions. The former includes postdoctoral researchers, as well as instructors, adjunct professors, non-tenured research professors, and staff scientists. Data about the latter are limited, but sources such as the Survey of Doctorate Recipients (SDR) suggest that the category likely encompasses a wide variety of positions across many employment sectors.

The declining probability of transitioning into an academic research position reflects the relatively flat job market in academia coupled with a growing supply of individuals trained in the biomedical sciences. Several factors contribute to the flat job market for early-career investigators. First, although the "number of bio-medical academic tenured/TT jobs did grow (by 150 percent, ~8,700 jobs) from 1981–2013," this increase could not keep pace with the "278 percent (102,000 people) increase in new U.S. Ph.D.s" (Kahn and Ginther, 2017, p. 92). Second, the abolition of mandatory retirement has allowed faculty to stay in their jobs longer, contingent on meeting performance expectations. A 2011 study of

---

[26] NSF. Survey of Doctorate Recipients. Employment trends from 1993 to 2013, calculated courtesy of Donna Ginther.

[27] See https://www.aamc.org/download/434462/data/june2015aib.pdf (accessed December 14, 2017).

full-time faculty members over age 60 found that 75 percent reported that they expected to work past "customary" retirement age, a shift that is reflected in the rising number of older investigators supported by NIH (National Academy of Sciences et al., 2014b). Between 1998 and 2014, the proportion of NIH-supported investigators over age 65 increased from 5 to 12 percent, while the percentage of investigators under age 50 declined from 54 to 39 percent (Figure 2-2).

A related factor contributing to the flat nature of the academic labor market is the considerable costs associated with recruiting a new faculty member, including startup packages that can exceed $1 million (Dorsey et al., 2009; Joiner, 2005). At the same time, the profit margins from clinical activity in academic health centers, which have traditionally been used to partially subsidize the research enterprise, are under increasing pressure. Further, public institutions have faced declining financial support from their state and local governments.

Physician-Scientists

One group of crucial contributors to biomedical research are physician-scientists—scientists with professional degrees[28] and training in clinical medicine who engage in biomedical research. As defined in the 2014 NIH Physician-Scientist Workforce Working Group Report (National Institutes of Health, 2014), physician-scientists typically engage in both clinical care and basic or clinical research, although not always at the same point in their career. The combination of training and experience allows the physician-scientist to contribute a unique perspective and affords them the opportunity to translate clinical observations to the laboratory to help identify the mechanisms of disease, as well as to apply the findings of basic science to patient care.

Physician-scientists also face challenges early in their research careers, including a lack of protected research time, loan repayment obligations, prolonged training, and a need for additional mentoring (National Institutes of Health, 2014). The 2014 NIH Physician-Scientist Workforce advisory committee estimated that about 1,000 physicians need to enter the research workforce each year to maintain the current physician-scientist workforce, but a significant number of physician-scientists move out of research when they are unable to renew their first NIH award (Dickler et al., 2007). NIH offers a variety of support mechanisms that are available to physician-scientists, such as the Loan Repayment Award (LRP), the Mentored Clinical Scientist Research Career Development Award (K08), the Career Transition Award (K22), the Pathway to Independence Award (K99/R00), and the Mentored Patient-Oriented Research Career Development Award (K23). However, certain pressures, including the increasing costs of obtaining a medical degree, the prolonged training period to develop clinical and research competen-

---

[28] As defined in the NIH Physician Scientist Workforce Report, these professional degrees include individuals with M.D., D.O., D.D.S./D.M.D., D.V.M./V.M.D., or nurses with research doctoral degrees.

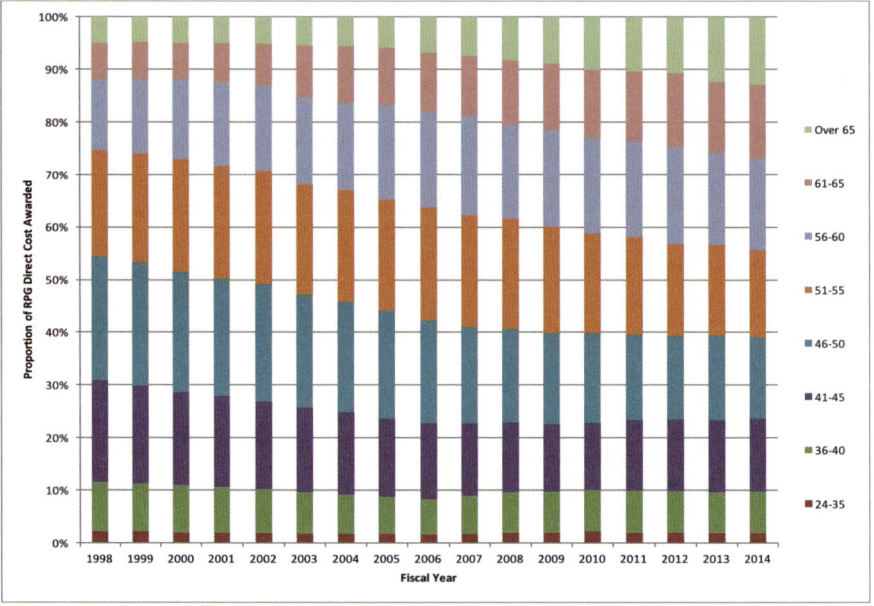

FIGURE 2-2 Proportion of NIH research project grant direct cost dollars awarded by age group.
SOURCE: Data and visualization from https://nexus.od.nih.gov/all/2015/03/25/age-of-investigator/ (accessed January 19, 2018).

cies, hospital funding pressures, and increasing clinical responsibilities, make it difficult for physician-scientists to pursue research.

Staff Scientists

A biomedical research career path that is drawing interest from across the biomedical research enterprise is that of staff, or "professional," scientists. Staff scientists[29] with Ph.D.'s provide essential functions as part of institutional core facilities or semi-permanent laboratory staff. They possess a full suite of research and analytical skills and often remain with research projects longer than graduate students and postdoctoral researchers. In some institutions, staff scientists can apply for their own federal research funding. A robust staff scientist path can offer investigators the promise of a sustainable academic research career outside of the traditional research faculty route, potentially easing the logjam of trainees waiting for such opportunities in postdoctoral positions. Written input from several professional societies, testimony to the committee, and statements from prominent

---

[29] See https://www.ncbi.nlm.nih.gov/pubmed/26625903 (accessed March 6, 2018).

scientists reveal a strong interest in providing support for more staff scientist positions. At the same time, additional research is needed to fully understand the potential impact of this population of researchers on the biomedical research ecosystem if the number of these positions were to grow.

Non-academic Research Positions

In 2013, slightly greater than 60 percent of biomedical Ph.D.'s in the United States worked outside of academia,[30] compared to slightly greater than 40 percent in 1993.[31] The pharmaceutical industry trains postdoctoral researchers in biological and behavioral sciences, who often transition into successful positions in the biopharmaceutical industry as group leaders, section heads, and distinguished scientist positions after their fellowships. To foster innovation, biopharmaceutical companies often collaborate with the government and the next generation of entrepreneurially minded basic and clinical science researchers through enterprises such as Small Business Innovation Research and Small Business Technology Transfer grants and the National Center for Advancing Translational Sciences.

The private sector also supports biomedical researchers through innovation health care accelerators and incubators such as StartUp Health and OneStart. Currently, several hundred state, national, and global networks of investors, partners, and customers who typically form peer networks provide financial support (i.e., direct funding and investment resources), education, mentoring, and coaching to promote the cutting edge of biomedical science.

One analysis of focus group responses suggests that personal values, combined with frustrations about long training periods, low postdoctoral researcher salaries, tight grant funding, and a highly competitive job market, have diminished biomedical scientists' interest in faculty research careers and has guided them toward non-academic careers (Gibbs and Griffin, 2013). However, as Figure 2-1 shows, the percentage of biomedical doctorates who are 1 to 5 years post degree attainment and are conducting research in non-academic positions has remained relatively steady between 1993 and 2013 (Figure 2-1). In contrast, the percentage of such doctorates in non-academic non-research positions has increased. More data are needed in this area to better understand the availability of and interest in non-academic research and non-research pathways.

---

[30] "Biomedical" here includes biological and health sciences, but because of the nature of the SDR this figure likely includes subfields previously excluded in other calculations in this chapter. NSF. Survey of Doctoral Recipients 2013, Table 42: Employed doctoral scientists and engineers, by occupation and sector of employment: 2013. https://ncsesdata.nsf.gov/doctoratework/2013/html/SDR2013_DST42.html (accessed February 2, 2018).

[31] NSF. Survey of Doctoral Recipients 1993, Table 20: Doctoral scientists and engineers, by field of doctorate and sector of employment: 1993. https://wayback.archive-it.org/5902/20160210235206/http://www.nsf.gov/statistics/s0893/dstable.htm (accessed February 2, 2018).

FUNDING FOR AN INDEPENDENT RESEARCH CAREER

For those postdoctoral researchers who hope to transition into academic research positions, access to research funding is crucial. That funding, however, is increasingly competitive. According to data provided by NIH, until the late 1990s, a newly hired assistant professor's first grant was most likely an NIH Type 1 (new) research project grant (R01) or equivalent award. The R01 is the flagship NIH RPG and remains an important benchmark for success on the path to independent research. Between 1998 and 2003, the NIH budget nearly doubled from roughly $13 billion to $27 billion ($21 billion in 1995 constant dollars) (Figure 2-3), and the success rate for type 1 competing R01-equivalent awards peaked at approximately 26 percent in 2000. However, the percentage of research awards to new investigators dropped steadily during those years, and, according to the 2005 National Academies *Bridges to Independence* report, it appears that "those with existing funding and established research programs received increased funding, in part to hire additional postdoctoral and graduate student researchers and further exacerbate the imbalance between trained researchers and available positions" (National Research Council, 2005, p. 40).

Since the doubling ended in 2004, NIH appropriations have declined in constant dollars, and the success rate for R01-equivalent awards has decreased rapidly for both established and new investigators[32] (Figure 2-3). The NIH budget received a supplemental bump in the American Recovery and Reinvestment Act (ARRA)[33] in 2009 and 2010, while sequestration in 2013 required a 5 percent ($1.55 billion) cut in the budget.[34]

The consequences of these significant funding changes can be compounded by the fact that NIH commits its funding to PIs in multi-year tranches—the average R01 grant is 3 to 5 years in duration, although funds are disbursed annually. At any given moment, close to 80 percent of NIH appropriations are committed to ongoing projects (Berg, 2016), with only the remainder available for new projects. Therefore, the size of the pool for new and competing projects in any given year is sensitive to year-to-year changes in the appropriation level. Between 1998 and 2006, the success rate for R01-equivalent awards for new investigators declined from 23 to 15 percent[35] (Figure 2-4).

One reason for the decline in success rates since 2004 is the change over time in the NIH budget. Another is the increase in the number of investigators seeking NIH funding each year. The number of applications for all NIH awards rose

---

[32] NIH defined "new investigators" as a program director/principal investigator (PD/PI) who has not previously competed successfully as a PD/PI for a substantial independent research award. https://grants.nih.gov/policy/early-investigators/index.htm (accessed January 19, 2018).

[33] See https://www.treasury.gov/initiatives/recovery/Pages/recovery-act.aspx.

[34] See https://www.nih.gov/news-events/news-releases/fact-sheet-impact-sequestration-national-institutes-health (accessed January 19, 2018).

[35] See https://report.nih.gov/NIHDatabook/Charts/Default.aspx?sid=1&index=0&catId=13&chartId=136 (accessed March 29, 2018).

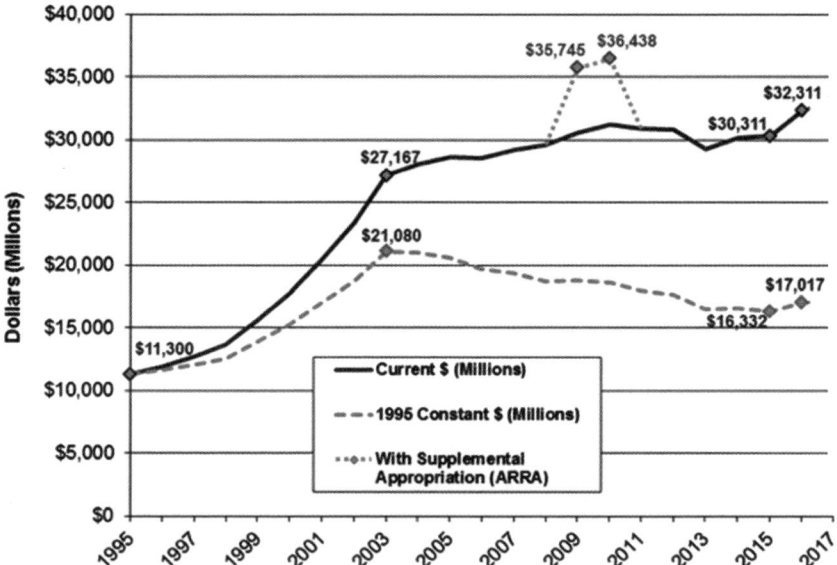

FIGURE 2-3 NIH appropriations in current and constant dollars, 1995-2017.
SOURCE: Adapted from http://www.faseb.org/Portals/2/PDFs/opa/2017/NIH%20Grants%20Slideshow.pptx.

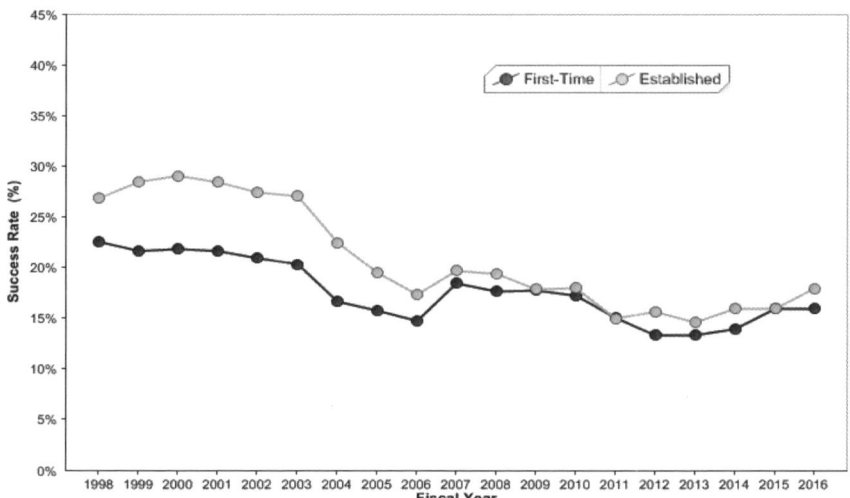

FIGURE 2-4 Success rates for competing type 1 R01 success rates for new and established investigators.
SOURCE: https://report.nih.gov/NIHDatabook/Charts/Default.aspx?showm=Y&chartId=136&catId=13 (accessed January 19, 2018).

steadily from 19,663 in 1998 to 41,420 in 2016 (Figure 2-5), while the number of applications for the Type 1 R01 awards increased by 97 percent for established investigators and 42 percent for new investigators.[36,37] In 2016, of more than 40,000 PIs that submitted competing RPG applications, only 11,434 (or 28%) received funding. Also that year, nearly 30,000 eligible biomedical investigators were unable to secure NIH funding to support their research (Figure 2-5), leading many to characterize the current biomedical ecosystem as "hypercompetitive," a situation with a stark imbalance between the dollars available for research and the expanding U.S. scientific community (Alberts et al., 2014; Fochler et al., 2016; Kamerlin, 2015; Kimble et al., 2015).

Faced with an increasing number of applicants for research awards—and concern about the ability of new investigators to compete for funding in that environment—NIH sought to boost support for new investigators by instituting a policy in fiscal year (FY)2007 to maintain comparable success rates for type 1 R01-equivalent applications from both experienced and new investigators.[38] NIH also established a policy that the majority of awarded new investigators should be early-stage investigators (ESIs),[39] defined as a "Program Director/Principal Investigator (PD/PI) who has completed their terminal research degree or end of post-graduate clinical training, whichever date is later, within the past 10 years and who has not previously competed successfully as PD/PI for a substantial NIH independent research award."[40] This new policy benefits both new investigators and ESIs by requiring peer reviewers to focus more on the proposed approach in grant applications than on an investigator's track record, and to expect less preliminary data than would be provided by established investigators.[41] NIH Institutes routinely fund ESI applications that score outside of the normal funding range by maintaining a separate payline for competing, investigator-initiated ESI R01 applications.[42] For example, in FY2017, the payline for ESI applications to

---

[36] NIH Data Book. Research and Training Grants: Competing Applications by Mechanism and Selected Activity Codes. https://report.nih.gov/nihdatabook/ (accessed February 2, 2018).

[37] See https://www.nih.gov/news-events/nih-research-grants-digital-press-kit (accessed January 19, 2018).

[38] See https://archives.nih.gov/asites/grants/08-22-2017/grants/guide/notice-files/NOT-OD-09-013.html (accessed December 15, 2017); https://archives.nih.gov/asites/grants/08-22-2017/grants/guide/notice-files/NOT-OD-07-030.html (accessed March 16, 2018).

[39] See https://grants.nih.gov/grants/guide/notice-files/NOT-OD-09-013.html (accessed February 8, 2018).

[40] See https://grants.nih.gov/policy/early-investigators/index.htm (accessed January 19, 2018).

[41] With the development of the Next Generation Researcher Initiative in 2017, NIH no longer uses the term new investigator and instead uses the term early-stage investigator (ESI).

[42] Since 2007, NIH Institutes and Centers (ICs) have maintained policies to guide enhanced funding for new investigators or ESIs. A recent Next Generation Researcher Initiative (NGRI) at NIH emphasized ESIs. However, grants from both new investigators and ESIs are still identified in eRAcommons (the online interface for NIH grants) and reviewed separately from grants from established investigators. An NIH NGRI advisory committee to the director and NIH ICs are currently discussing final recommendations on policies to enhance independence and research funding for early-stage and new researchers.

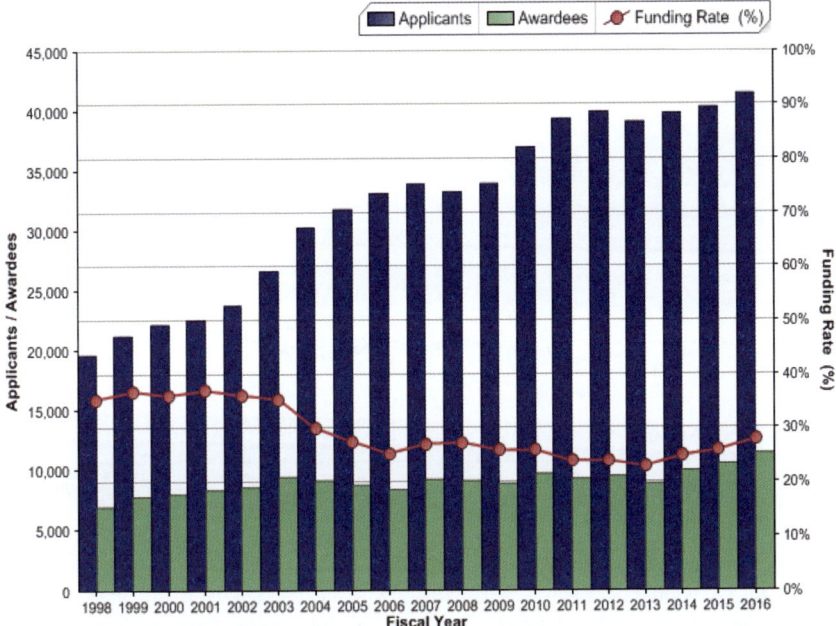

FIGURE 2-5 Individual applicants, awardees, and funding rates of NIH research project grants.
SOURCE: Data from NIH Data Book. https://report.nih.gov/NIHDatabook/Charts/Default.aspx?showm=Y&chartId=164&catId=13 (accessed January 19, 2018).

the National Heart, Lung, and Blood Institute (NHLBI) was set at 10 percentile points above the regular R01 payline.[43]

This new investigator policy went into effect in FY2007, and the number of new investigator R01 awardees increased slightly between 2008 and 2010 (Figure 2-6)[44] (these data exclude awards made from the ARRA in 2009 and 2010). However, in 2013, the number of new investigator awardees dipped to 2005 levels, which coincided with budget sequestration. NIH estimated that sequestration resulted in approximately 640 fewer RPG awardees compared to FY2012, but it is unclear how new investigators and ESIs were affected.[45] Since sequestration,

---

[43] See https://www.nhlbi.nih.gov/research/funding/general/current-operating-guidelines (accessed December 15, 2017).

[44] See https://report.nih.gov/NIHDatabook/Charts/Default.aspx?showm=YandchartId=168andcatId=22 (accessed December 15, 2017).

[45] NIH. Fact Sheet: Impact of Sequestration on the National Institutes of Health. https://www.nih.gov/news-events/news-releases/fact-sheet-impact-sequestration-national-institutes-health (accessed December 15, 2017).

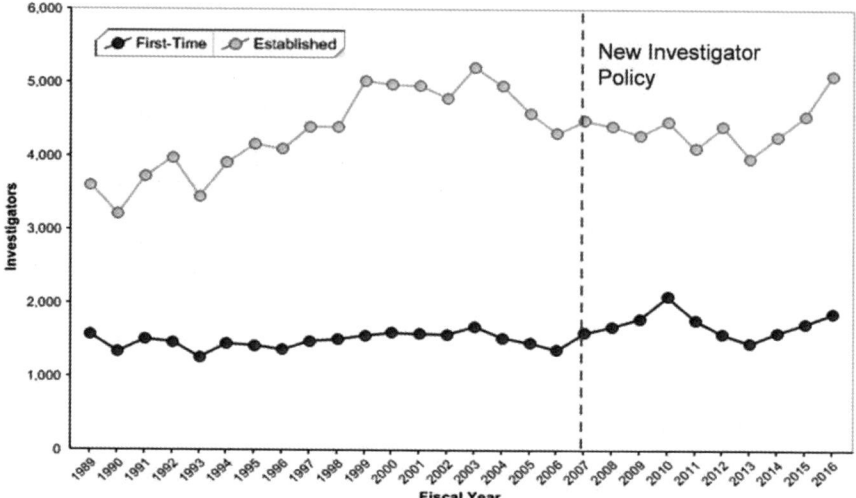

FIGURE 2-6 Number of investigators supported by NIH R01-equivalent awards by career stage.
SOURCE: Data and visualization from NIH Data Book. https://report.nih.gov/NIHDatabook/Charts/Default.aspx?showm=Y&chartId=168&catId=22 (accessed February 8, 2018).

the number of new investigators awarded R01-equivalents has increased, but not as rapidly as for established investigators.

Although NIH's new investigator policy leveled success rates between new and established investigators and temporarily boosted the number of new investigators receiving R01-equivalent awards, the average age of first receipt of an R01-equivalent award rose from 39.3 in 1990 to 44.2 in 2016.[46] This increase applies across Ph.D.'s (from 38.9 to 43.3), M.D.'s (from 39.9 to 46.5), and M.D.-Ph.D.'s (from 40.2 to 45.9) (Figure 2-7). In addition, the number of NIH-supported researchers under age 46 has declined over a 32-year period,[47] even after implementation of new investigator and ESI policies.[48]

The precise reason for why the age of receipt of the first NIH R01-equivalent award has increased, even as the success rate of new investigators relative to

---

[46] Data provided courtesy of NIH.
[47] See https://www.nap.edu/catalog/11249/bridges-to-independence-fostering-the-independence-of-new-investigators-in (accessed January 19, 2018).
[48] See https://grants.nih.gov/grants/guide/notice-files/NOT-OD-08-121.html.

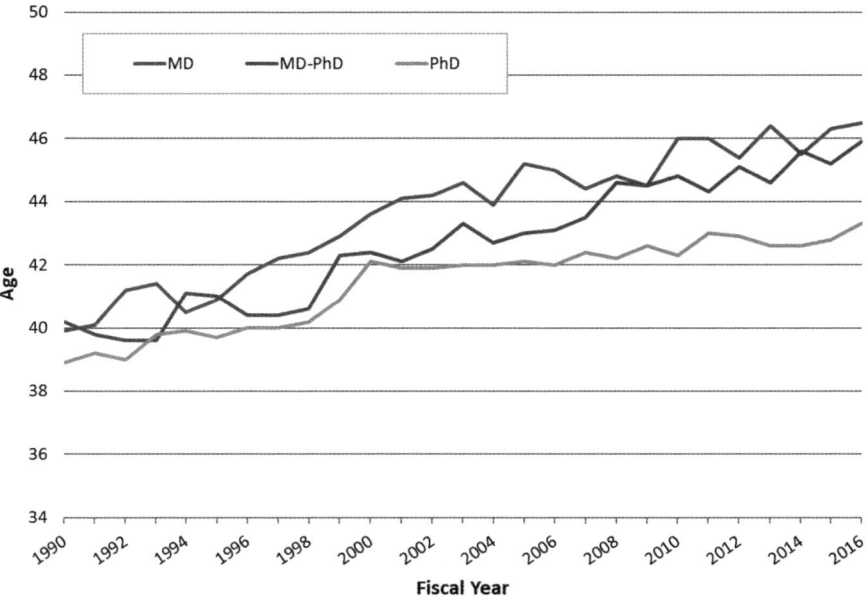

FIGURE 2-7 Age at first-R01 equivalent by degree type.
SOURCE: Data provided courtesy of NIH.

established investigators has stabilized, is unclear and a matter of debate.[49] NIH data show that the number of years to first R01 since the investigator's last degree has increased over time as well, suggesting that the increase in the age at first R01 cannot be explained by any delays in the start or culmination of doctoral education (Figure 2-8). The data also show that the number of years on average between an investigator's first R01 and second R01 has mostly held steady over time, suggesting that whatever is causing the delays over time in the capacity of investigators to obtain their first R01 is largely confined to the pursuit of that first grant (Figure 2-9). Finally, the rise in the age exists across NIH Institutes, which suggests an effect of larger workforce trends that apply across all areas of biomedical research (Figure 2-10). The rise persists across race[50] and gender[51] as well.

---

[49] Many researchers consider the phenomenon of investigators delaying retirement, and therefore continuing to compete with new investigators in the NIH pool, as one leading factor (Heggenness et al., 2017; Levitt and Levitt, 2017).

[50] From 1990 to 2016, the age at first R01-equivalent for white, Asian, and multi-race investigators increased from 39.1 to 44.1, while the age for underrepresented minorities increased from 38.9 to 43.3. Data provided courtesy of NIH.

[51] From 1990 to 2016, the age at first R01-equivalent for female investigators increased from 39.7 to 44.2, while the age for male investigators increased from 39.1 to 44.2. Data provided courtesy of NIH.

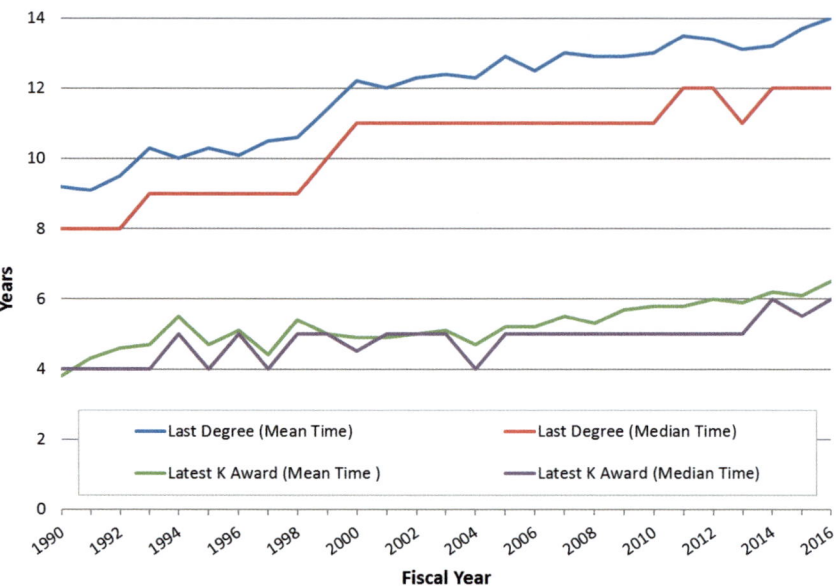

FIGURE 2-8 Years to first R01-equivalent award since last degree award.
SOURCE: Data provided courtesy of NIH.

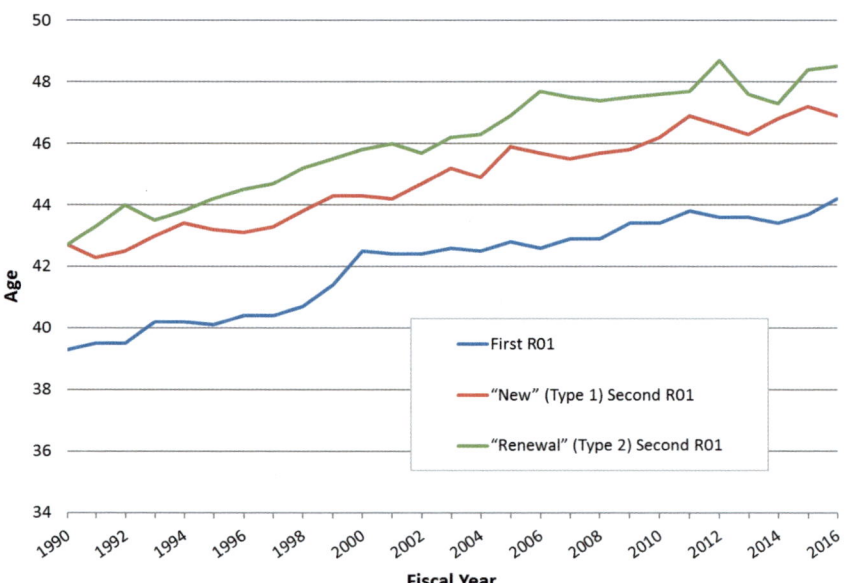

FIGURE 2-9 Average age over time to first R01, new (type 1) second R01, and renewal (type 2) second R01.
SOURCE: Data provided courtesy of NIH.

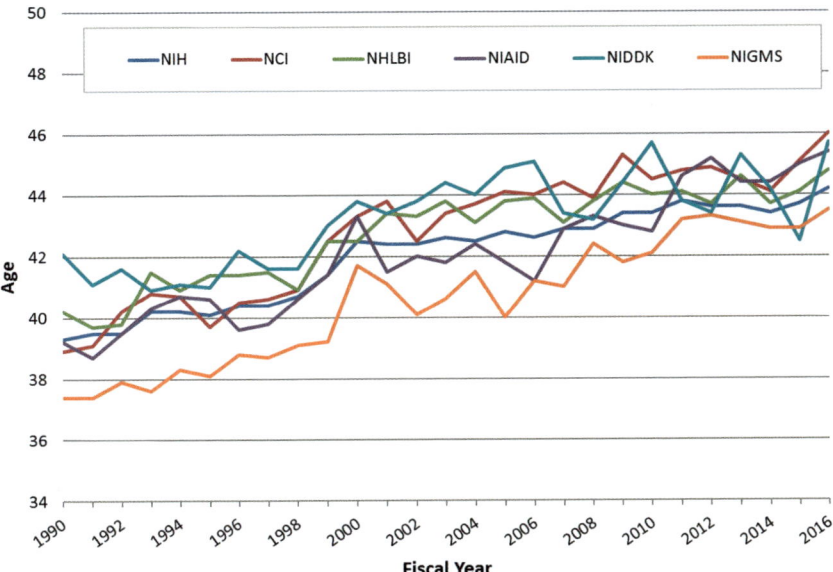

FIGURE 2-10 Age at first R01-equivalent award by NIH Institute.
SOURCE: Data provided courtesy of NIH.

Today, even when ESIs and new investigators do receive an R01-equivalent award, they often confront the challenge of the declining purchasing power of these awards, because the size of these awards has not tracked with either overall inflation or the rising cost of conducting research as measured by the Biomedical Research and Development Price Index,[52] despite some increase in the average costs for R01s when adjusted for inflation. As a result, investigators often need to secure more than one source of financial support to establish and sustain their laboratories.

Additional avenues of federal research support for emerging biomedical researchers include NIH's Exploratory/Developmental Research Grant Award (R21), NIH Director's New Innovator Award (DP2), Early Independence Award (DP5), and Pathway to Independence Award (K99/R00). According to NIH, the non-renewable R21 grant mechanism, as opposed to the renewable R01 award, is intended to encourage exploratory or developmental research by providing support for the early and conceptual stages of project development, usually defined as lasting no longer than 2 years. Although R21 awards are not specifically designed to support ESIs, data provided by NIH highlights the fact that the R01 is increasingly giving way to the R21 and other awards as the research grant that starts investiga-

---

[52] See https://officeofbudget.od.nih.gov/gbipriceindexes.html (accessed January 19, 2018).

tors' NIH-funded career (Figure 2-11). Each year, roughly the same number of investigators now apply for an R21 and an R01 as their first grant.[53] These trends are observed across all age cohorts.[54]

R21 awards may be regarded as an opportunity to secure initial funding for an emerging investigator's independent research career, but analysis of R21 awardees shows that receipt of the award does not increase the success rate for receiving an R01-equivalent award.[55] Not all individual NIH Institutes offer R21 awards, and data provided by NIH show that applications for R21 awards have increased to the point where success rates for receiving the award are now lower than for R01-equivalent awards, at 15 percent and 20 percent, respectively, in 2016.[56] In addition, R21 awards provide less funding over a shorter time period compared to R01-equivalent awards, and thus are less ideal for establishing an independent research career. The combined budget for direct costs for the 2-year R21 project period may not exceed $275,000, and no more than $150,000 may be requested in any single year.[57] In 2016, the average cost of competing R21 awards was $221,434, whereas the average cost for an R01 award, which can span 5 years, was $476,631 per year.[58] The higher level of funding and longer funding period for R01 grants are designed to provide researchers with the time and resources necessary to collect and publish data that represent a substantial addition to biomedical knowledge.

The NIH Director's New Innovator Award (DP2) program offers a small number of awards through the NIH Common Fund to support highly innovative research from promising ESIs. DP2 applicants can request up to $1.5 million in direct costs spread over the 5-year grant period. Data on the DP2 awards indicate that awardees have a higher rate of application for R01 awards compared to a matched cohort of ESIs who receive R01 awards, although DP2 awardees are not more successful at receiving an R01 award (National Institutes of Health, 2017). Although the DP2 award seems to be an important mechanism for supporting ESIs as they transition into research independence, NIH expects to make only 33 awards in 2018, depending on availability of funds in the NIH Common Fund. This represents a decrease from the 55 awards in 2017.[59]

Developed in response to the National Academies *Bridges to Independence* report (National Research Council, 2005), NIH launched the K99/R00 Pathway to Independence awards in 2006 to

---

[53] Data provided courtesy of NIH.

[54] Data provided courtesy of NIH.

[55] Open Mike Blog. R01 and R21 Applications and Awards: Trends and Relationships Across NIH. https://nexus.od.nih.gov/all/2016/11/04/nih-r01-r21/ (accessed February 8, 2018).

[56] See https://report.nih.gov/NIHDatabook/Charts/Default.aspx?showm=Yandchartld=202andcatld=2 (accessed February 9, 2018).

[57] See https://grants.nih.gov/grants/funding/funding_program.htm (accessed January 19, 2018).

[58] See https://report.nih.gov/NIHDatabook/Charts/Default.aspx?showm=Yandchartld=294andcatld=2 (accessed February 8, 2018).

[59] See https://commonfund.nih.gov/newinnovator/faq (accessed December 15, 2017).

THE LANDSCAPE FOR THE NEXT GENERATION OF RESEARCHERS 41

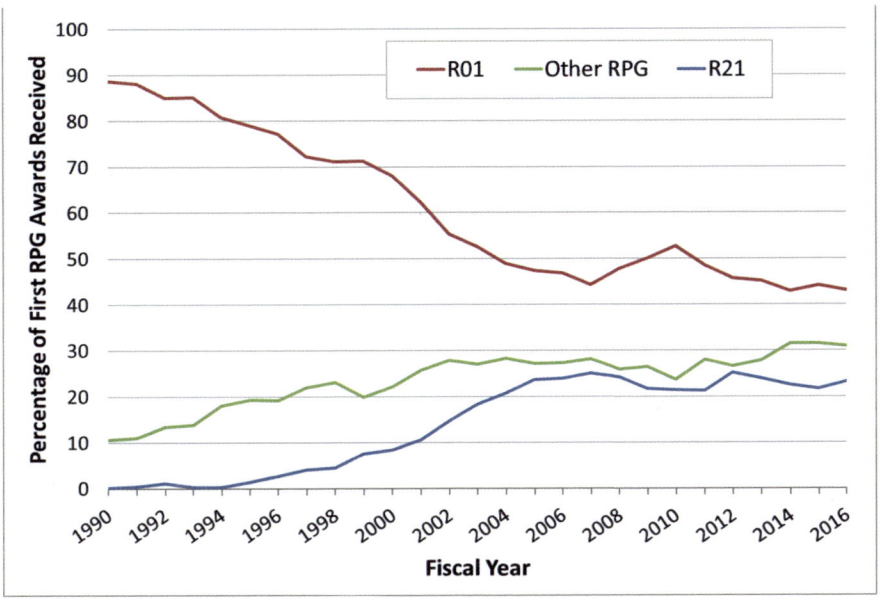

FIGURE 2-11 First competing research project grant award received by investigators.
NOTE: Other RPGs for purposes of this figure include a range of R-series, DP-series, P-series, and U-series awards.
SOURCE: Data provided courtesy of NIH.

... help outstanding postdoctoral researchers with a research and/or clinical doctorate degree complete needed, mentored career development and transition in a timely manner to independent, tenure-track, or equivalent faculty positions. The K99/R00 award is intended to foster the development of a creative, independent research program that will be competitive for subsequent independent funding and that will help advance the mission of the NIH.[60]

The K99/R00 award is unique among NIH awards in that it combines an initial mentored phase—a K99-supported postdoctoral position—with the investigator's first independent research support, the R00 phase. This award is available to individuals who have less than 4 years of postdoctoral training, and to non-U.S. citizens and physician-scientists. The K99 phase lasts a maximum of 2 years, and the R00 phase provides up to 3 years of independent research support for individuals who have secured an independent, tenure-track, or equivalent faculty position by the end of the K99 period. In 2016, 231 K99s were awarded

---

[60] See https://grants.nih.gov/grants/guide/pa-files/PA-16-077.html (accessed December 15, 2017).

with a success rate of 23 percent.[61] One recent analysis of the K99/R00 award reveals that recipients have a higher success rate for subsequent R01 and other grants compared to those supported on other K-series career development awards (Carlson et al., 2016).

Additional support for ESIs from NIH includes several innovative Institute-specific programs that seek to support these researchers' transition to independence: the National Institute of Mental Health (NIMH) Biobehavioral Research Awards for Innovative New Scientists (BRAINS) award, the National Institute of General Medical Sciences (NIGMS) Maximizing Investigators' Research Award (MIRA), and the NIH Director's Early Independence Award (DP5). Together, these programs fund only 100 or so awards per year.[62]

The number of federal research awards to help investigators transition into independent faculty research positions is limited, and postdoctoral researchers are typically not prepared or, often even eligible,[63] to submit an R01 application prior to obtaining a faculty appointment. Funding for emerging investigators is generally provided by their host institutions, and universities have reported surges in the size of start-up packages offered to junior faculty. In testimony to the committee, committee member Nancy Andrews, former dean and vice chancellor for academic affairs at Duke University School of Medicine, confirmed this phenomenon: she observed that the current "range for the amount of cash that basic science department assistant professors are offered is probably between about $800,000 and the highest I have heard is $3.5 million nationally . . . but more typically it would be something like $1.2 to $1.8 million, sometimes including three years of salary." These trends align with data revealing that higher education institutions are the second largest funder of basic science research in this country behind the government (Figure 2-12). This upward pressure may make K99/R00 award recipients more attractive for recruitment to faculty positions at academic institutions because they have been successful at obtaining NIH funding.

OTHER CHALLENGES IN PURSUING RESEARCH CAREERS

Funding remains the paramount concern for early-career scientists, but a 2016 survey of *Nature* readers highlighted additional areas of concern (Powell, 2016). Of the nearly 12,000 readers who responded to the survey question, "What do you think is the biggest challenge facing early-career scientists?", the top concerns included not only securing research funding but also balancing work and home responsibilities and navigating the publishing culture. Reports that scientists find themselves spending more time writing grant applications and less time

---

[61] NIH Data Book. Research Project Grants: Competing Applications, Awards, and Success Rates. https://report.nih.gov/nihdatabook/ (accessed February 2, 2018).

[62] See https://grants.nih.gov/grants/guide/rfa-files/RFA-RM-17-008.html and https://loop.nigms.nih.gov/2016/08/first-mira-awards-to-new-and-early-stage-investigators/ (accessed January 19, 2018).

[63] Eligibility restrictions often apply to the institution.

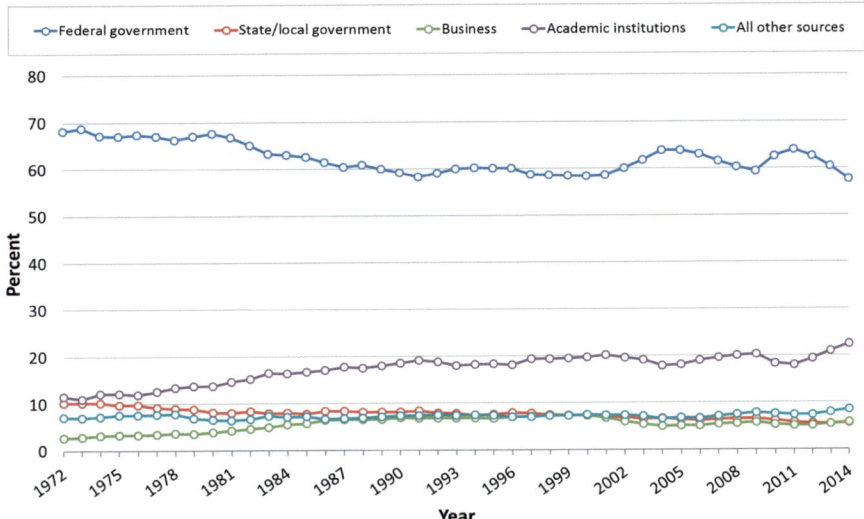

FIGURE 2-12 Academic science and engineering research and development expenditures, by source of funding.
NOTE: Academic institutions' funds exclude research funds spent from multipurpose accounts.
SOURCE: Adapted from https://www.nsf.gov/statistics/2016/nsb20161/#/report/chapter-5/expenditures-and-funding-for-academic-r-d (accessed January 19, 2018).

doing creative research are borne out by data showing that young investigators are submitting a larger number of grant applications each year than ever before.[64] Nearly two-thirds of the survey respondents also said they considered quitting research at some point in their career, and, in fact, it appears that investigators today are leaving the NIH-funded workforce at an accelerated rate relative to the past (Figure 2-13).[65]

---

[64] See http://www.unitedformedicalresearch.com/wp-content/uploads/2012/07/Broken-Pipeline.pdf. Data provided courtesy of NIH show that applicants ages 36 to 45 submitted an average of 3.42 grant applications each between 2011 and 2016, an average of 3.11 grant applications each between 2004 and 2010, an average of 2.59 grant applications each between 1998 and 2003 (during the doubling), and an average of 2.98 grant application each from 1990 to 1997. This same trend can be seen in each of the other age cohorts as well.

[65] The figure shows data for PIs who received an NIH RPG. Data provided courtesy of NIH also suggest a similar trend for investigators who never obtained an RPG. A greater percentage (58 percent) of investigators who first applied for an RPG during 2004-2010 have failed to receive any funding than investigators who first applied for an RPG during the NIH doubling from 1998 to 2003 (48 percent) or 1990 to 1997 (53 percent). These results are tempered by the fact that investigators from 2004 to 2010 are more likely than earlier cohorts to yet obtain funding at some point in the future.

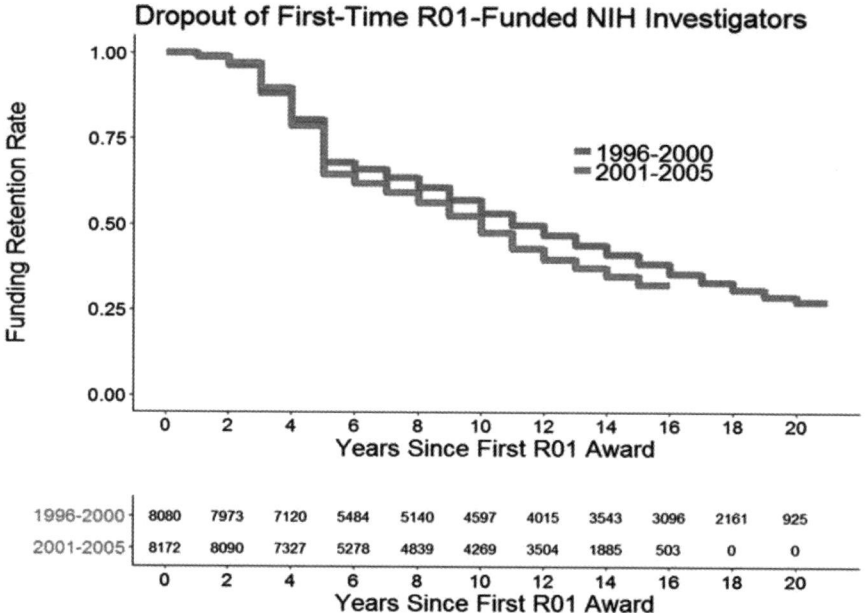

FIGURE 2-13 Dropout of first-time R01-funded NIH investigators.
NOTE: Plot shows PI retention rate by years since first R01-equivalent award. Each curve shows dropout (conversely, retention) of investigators after they received their first R01-equivalent award. Investigators are grouped into cohorts based on the first fiscal year of their first R01-equivalent award.
SOURCE: Chart provided courtesy of NIH.

Of special concern for the biomedical research enterprise are the enduring barriers to independent faculty research careers faced by women and individuals from underrepresented racial and ethnic groups. As of 2016, women had equivalent NIH RPG success rates and representation in NIH research career development awards as their male counterparts,[66] yet the average total research grant size for men was nearly $75,000 more than for women.[67] Additionally, faculty positions are often required for eligibility to apply for an NIH grant, but between 2011 and 2012, women represented only 30 percent of biomedical faculty at the assistant, associate, and full professor levels (Valantine et

---

[66] Research Career Development Award Recipients and Kirschstein-NRSA Trainees and Fellows: Representation of Women, by Activity and Career Stage. https://report.nih.gov/NIHDatabook/Charts/Default.aspx?sid=0andindex=1andcatId=15andchartId=170 (accessed February 9, 2018).

[67] Research Grants: Average Size, by Gender. https://report.nih.gov/NIHDatabook/Charts/Default.aspx?showm=YandchartId=173andcatId=15 (accessed February 9, 2018).

al., 2016). In fact, women represented only 32 percent of all NIH-supported investigators on RPGs.[68]

It is unclear whether the high rate of attrition for women between Ph.D. attainment and faculty research positions is due to personal choice or hiring discrimination, but the 2007 National Academies report *Beyond Bias and Barriers* reported that women leave academia because of a lack of mentorship or guidance and difficulty managing family and career responsibilities, among many other socially and culturally influenced factors (National Academy of Sciences et al., 2007). These findings are consistent with those from a 2009 study that revealed that female Ph.D.'s with children, or planning to have children, opted out of the NIH R01 pool in favor of a career they believed would be more compatible with their family work-life plans (Ginther and Kahn, 2006).

Despite longstanding efforts to increase racial and ethnic diversity in the biomedical research workforce, the proportion of individuals from underrepresented minority groups hired into faculty research positions and securing NIH RPGs has not matched their steady gains in Ph.D. attainment (Gibbs et al., 2016). A recent analysis by Meyers et al. (2018) examining underrepresented minority research faculty participation at medical schools reveals significant retention issues between their postdoctoral experiences and faculty research positions. Once in faculty research positions, African Americans applicants experience significant disparities in R01-funding (Ginther et al., 2011). Additionally, African Americans proportionately resubmit fewer R01 applications than do White, Asian, or Hispanic applicants (National Institutes of Health, 2012b). In an analysis spanning 1999 to 2009, 73 percent of applications from African Americans were not discussed in NIH peer review, which may have impacted their resubmission rates (National Institutes of Health, 2012b). The decreased representation of underrepresented minority biomedical postdoctoral and faculty researchers coincides with a decline in NIH-supported training and career development programs with a focus on diversity and remains an area of continued concern (Valantine et al., 2016).

The challenges facing early-career biomedical researchers command urgent and sustained attention. In a *Nature* article, Jon Lorsch, head of NIGMS, said that the 2016 *Nature* survey results echo what he hears from early-career scientists as he travels nationwide: "We risk losing a generation of researchers at the prime of their creativity and energy" (Powell, 2016).

REFERENCES

Alberts, B., M. W. Kirschner, S. Tilghman, and H. Varmus. 2014. Rescuing US biomedical research from its systemic flaws. *Proceedings of the National Academy of Sciences of the United States of America* 111(16):5773-5777.

---

[68] Research Grant Investigators: Representation of Women, by Mechanism. https://report.nih.gov/NIHDatabook/Charts/Default.aspx?showm=YandchartId=169andcatId=15 (accessed February 9, 2018).

American Academy of Arts and Sciences. 2014. *Restoring the foundation: The vital role of research in preserving the American dream.* Cambridge, MA: American Academy of Arts and Sciences.

Berg, J. 2016. Modeling the annual number of new and competing NIH research project grants. In *ScienceHound.* Washington, DC: American Association for the Advancement of Science.

Carlson, D. E., W. C. Wang, and J. D. Scott. 2016. Initial outcomes for the NHLBI K99/R00 pathway to independence program in relation to long-standing career development programs: Implications for trainees, mentors, and institutions. *Circulation Research* 119(8):904-908.

Dickler, H. B., D. Fang, S. J. Heinig, E. Johnson, and D. Korn. 2007. New physician-investigators receiving National Institutes of Health research project grants: A historical perspective on the "endangered species." *JAMA* 297(22):2496-2501.

Dorsey, E. R., B. C. Van Wuyckhuyse, C. A. Beck, W. P. Passalacqua, and D. S. Guzick. 2009. Economics of new faculty hires in basic science. *Academic Medicine: Journal of the Association of American Medical Colleges* 84(1):26-31.

FASEB (Federation of American Societies for Experimental Biology). 2015. *Sustaining discovery in biological and medical sciences: A framework for discussion.* Bethesda, MD: Federation of American Societies for Experimental Biology.

Fochler, M., U. Felt, and R. Müller. 2016. Unsustainable growth, hyper-competition, and worth in life science research: Narrowing evaluative repertoires in doctoral and postdoctoral scientists' work and lives. *Minerva* 54(2):175-200.

Gibbs, K. D., J. Basson, I. M. Xierali, and D. A. Broniatowski. 2016. Decoupling of the minority PhD talent pool and assistant professor hiring in medical school basic science departments in the US. *Elife* 5.

Gibbs, K. D., Jr., and K. A. Griffin. 2013. What do I want to be with my PhD? The roles of personal values and structural dynamics in shaping the career interests of recent biomedical science PhD graduates. *CBE Life Sciences Education* 12(4):711-723.

Gibbs, K. D., J. McGready, and K. Griffin. 2015. Career development among American biomedical postdocs. *CBE Life Sciences Education* 14(4):ar44.

Ginther, D. K., W. T. Schaffer, J. Schnell, B. Masimore, F. Liu, L. L. Haak, and R. Kington. 2011. Race, ethnicity, and NIH research awards. *Science* 333(6045):1015-1019.

Ginther, D. K., and S. Kahn. 2006. *Does science promote women? Evidence from academia 1973-2001.* Cambridge, MA: National Bureau of Economic Researh.

Heggeness, M. L., K. T. Gunsalus, J. Pacas, and G. McDowell. 2017. The new face of US science. *Nature* 541(7635):21-23.

Institute of Medicine, National Academy of Sciences, and National Academy of Engineering. 2000. *Enhancing the postdoctoral experience for scientists and engineers: A guide for postdoctoral scholars, advisers, institutions, funding organizations, and disciplinary societies.* Washington, DC: The National Academies Press.

Joiner, K. A. 2005. A strategy for allocating central funds to support new faculty recruitment. *Academic Medicine* 80(3):218-224.

Kahn, S., and D. K. Ginther. 2017. The impact of postdoctoral training on early careers in biomedicine. *Nature Biotechnology* 35(1):90-94.

Kamerlin, S. C. 2015. Hypercompetition in biomedical research evaluation and its impact on young scientist careers. *International Microbiology* 18(4):253-261.

Kimble, J., W. M. Bement, Q. Chang, B. L. Cox, N. R. Drinkwater, R. L. Gourse, A. A. Hoskins, A. Huttenlocher, P. K. Kreeger, P. F. Lambert, M. R. Mailick, S. Miyamoto, R. L. Moss, K. M. O'Connor-Giles, A. Roopra, K. Saha, and H. S. Seidel. 2015. Strategies from UW-Madison for rescuing biomedical research in the US. *Elife* 4:e09305.

Levitt, M., and J. Levitt. 2017. Future of fundamental discovery in US biomedical research. *Proceedings of the National Academy of Sciences of the United States of America* 114(25):6498-6503.

McDowell, G. S., K. T. Gunsalus, D. C. MacKellar, S. A. Mazzilli, V. P. Pai, P. R. Goodwin, E. M. Walsh, A. Robinson-Mosher, T. A. Bowman, J. Kraemer, M. L. Erb, E. Schoenfeld, L. Shokri, J. D. Jackson, A. Islam, M. D. Mattozzi, K. A. Krukenberg, and J. K. Polka. 2014. Shaping the future of research: A perspective from junior scientists. *F1000Res* 3:291.

Meyers, L. C., A. M. Brown, L. Moneta-Koehler, and R. Chalkley. 2018. Survey of checkpoints along the pathway to diverse biomedical research faculty. PLoS ONE 13(1):e0190606.

National Academy of Sciences, National Academy of Engineering, and Institute of Medicine. 2014a. *The postdoctoral experience revisited*. Washington, DC: The National Academies Press.

National Academy of Sciences, National Academy of Engineering, and Institute of Medicine. 2014b. *The arc of the academic research career: Issues and implications for U.S. science and engineering leadership: Summary of a workshop*. Washington, DC: The National Academies Press.

National Academy of Sciences, National Academy of Engineering, and Institute of Medicine. 2007. *Beyond bias and barriers: Fulfilling the potential of women in academic science and engineering*. Washington, DC: The National Academies Press.

National Institutes of Health. 2014. *National Institutes of Health Physician-Scientist Workforce Working Group report*. Bethesda, MD: National Institutes of Health.

National Institutes of Health. 2012a. *Biomedical Research Workforce Working Group report*. Bethesda, MD: National Institutes of Health.

National Institutes of Health. 2012b. *Draft report of the Advisory Committee to the Director Working Group on Diversity in the Biomedical Research Workforce*. Bethesda, MD: The National Institutes of Health.

National Institutes of Health. 2017. *National Institutes of Health Director's New Innovator Award outcomes evaluation*. Bethesda, MD: The National Institutes of Health.

National Research Council. 2011. *Research training in the biomedical, behavioral, and clinical research sciences*. Washington, DC: The National Academies Press.

National Research Council. 2005. *Bridges to independence: Fostering the independence of new investigators in biomedical research*. Washington, DC: The National Academies Press.

Powell, K. 2016. Young, talented and fed-up: Scientists tell their stories. *Nature* 538(7626):446-449.

Sauermann, H., and M. Roach. 2016. Scientific workforce. Why pursue the postdoc path? *Science* 352(6286):663-664.

Sauermann, H., and M. Roach. 2012. Science PhD career preferences: Levels, changes, and advisor encouragement. *PloS One* 7(5):e36307.

Valantine, H. A., P. K. Lund, and A. E. Gammie. 2016. From the NIH: A systems approach to increasing the diversity of the biomedical research workforce. *CBE Life Sciences Education* 15(3).

3

Transparency, Shared Responsibility, and Sustainability

The genesis of this report stems from concerns expressed by members of Congress that the nation's emerging biomedical[1] researchers face unprecedented, systemic challenges that limit their ability to begin and sustain their careers as independent investigators. As Chapter 1 argues and the data presented in Chapter 2 show, those concerns are well-founded. This and the following chapters present recommendations reflecting the committee's strong view that addressing these challenges and creating a better path forward for the nation's emerging biomedical researchers is not the sole responsibility of the National Institutes of Health (NIH), but is rather a shared responsibility of stakeholders throughout the entire biomedical research enterprise.

SHARED RESPONSIBILITY

The American biomedical research enterprise is a complex ecosystem that includes a range of public and private stakeholders with overlapping and sometimes conflicting interests, objectives, and incentives. The decisions of many of these stakeholders cannot help but affect the way in which the next generation of investigators are recruited into the system. For an enterprise dependent upon identifying, training, and recruiting a cadre of investigators, few well-established forums exist to consistently evaluate and discuss the consequences of widely distributed and seemingly unconnected decisions by these different stakeholders. Mainly, stakeholder engagement on the issues facing the biomedical research

---

[1] In this report, "biomedical" refers to the full range of biological, biomedical, behavioral, and health sciences supported by the National Institutes of Health.

enterprise—including those affecting young investigators—has been episodic and uncoordinated.

When and where it has occurred, engagement has taken the form of working groups, advisory councils, and ad hoc committees such as this one. These bodies have produced no shortage of recommendations addressed to different stakeholders in the biomedical research system, such as federal funding agencies, research institutions, professional societies, private-sector organizations, principal investigators, and the young researchers themselves. These endeavors, however, tend to be sporadic and discrete, and thus do not maintain sustained stewardship of the enterprise. These advisory bodies usually disband after issuing their recommendations, so there is no sustained oversight or collaboration on what occurs afterwards. Those advisory bodies that do meet regularly—such as advisory councils at NIH—are designed principally to advise the federal government on its own functioning and decisions, rather than to serve as a venue for the multilateral exchange of ideas and information that bear on the responsibilities of everyone in the ecosystem. There is little in the way of regular, ongoing, and shared conversations among these stakeholders about how best to implement recommendations and advance common interests that benefit the entire biomedical research system (Daniels, 2015). Assessment of responses to prior recommendations (Appendix B) illustrates that NIH has been responsive to calls for action, but NIH is not, nor should be, the sole driver of efforts to support the next generation of researchers.

The committee, therefore, has concluded that the need exists for an umbrella coordinating body to serve as an ongoing, independent forum for analyzing and addressing challenges confronting the biomedical workforce in a sustained manner, and to monitor implementation of the recommendations set forth in this and other reports. This body would include representatives from research universities, nonprofit advocacy associations, disciplinary societies, industry, NIH, and other federal agencies.

A number of other areas of national policy priority that exhibit a close integration of public and private actors and a need for engaged action across a sector have benefited from standing multi-stakeholder bodies that promote the ongoing exchange of information and ensure sustained oversight of strategic initiatives. Examples include the protection of critical infrastructure,[2] standards-setting,[3] and

---

[2] For example, Infragard is a network of 501(c)(3)—developed in the wake of Presidential Decision Direction 63 on critical infrastructure protection, and originally managed out of the National Infrastructure Protection Center and includes members from the Federal Bureau of Investigations, state law enforcement agencies, academia, other government agencies, business and other organizations, and was created to provide formal and informal channels to promote the exchange of information about how to protect our nation's critical infrastructures and key resources.

[3] The American National Standards Institute is a 501(c)(3) not-for-profit organization composed of government agencies, companies, academic and international bodies, and others that seeks to facilitate voluntary consensus standards and conformity assessment systems and to safeguard their integrity.

the interoperability of emergent technologies.[4] Each of these bodies is structured in a somewhat different way, and serves a somewhat different purpose, but common among them is a diverse membership across public and private stakeholders in service of a common goal, and a recognition that earlier siloed approaches to decision-making were inadequate to the challenges at hand.

The time has arrived to create a similar coordinating council for the biomedical research enterprise—to serve as a consultative forum for analyzing and addressing issues confronting the biomedical workforce, assembling information and resources across the sector, monitoring implementation and assessing the impact of the recommendations set forth in this report, and developing and overseeing new initiatives in an ongoing manner. The committee recommends the establishment of the Biomedical Research Enterprise Council (BREC) to serve as this forum.

Although the committee does not want to be too prescriptive in the structure of the BREC, because it expects the council will both want and need space to grow and adapt as needed over time, its success will depend in no small measure on decisions regarding its funding and membership. The committee comments briefly on both below.

Launching the BREC

The committee recommends that the BREC be an independent not-for-profit organization, to ensure that it can play a stewardship role on behalf of the full range of stakeholders. However, the committee recognizes that the first few years after the BREC launches will be critical in establishing its stability, trajectory, and sustainability. Therefore, the committee recommends that NIH play a temporarily outsized role in financing the BREC in its earliest stages. The committee expects that responsibility for support of the BREC soon thereafter will transition to the broader biomedical community (with some continuing support from NIH).

The committee notes that a number of current examples of independent public-private bodies started their existence under the close sponsorship of a federal agency before transitioning to self-support.[5] In addition, there are now bodies supported initially by a federal agency, with the expectation that they would transition to self-support. For example, the Department of Energy formed the Gridwise Architecture Council (GWAC)—an entity with public and private membership that seeks to advance interoperability among the entities that interact

---

[4] The Smart Grid Interoperability Panel is a 501(c)(3) not-for-profit organization, originally launched by the National Institute of Standards and Technology (NIST), that coordinates standards development for the smart grid and brings together public and private stakeholders to interact and accelerate standards harmonization and to advance the interoperability of smart electric grid devices and systems.

[5] See, e.g., *supra* note 2, Infragard managed out of NIPC); note 4 (Smart Grid Interoperability started originally in NIST).

with the nation's electric power system, and continues to provide the GWAC with administrative and logistical support, but "operational assistance is expected to eventually transition to related industry organizations."[6] The committee notes that this and similar bodies do not set an exact precedent for the BREC, but have succeeded under a sequenced model of public funding followed by broader support that balances the need for early support and stability and long-term independence.

The committee does not expect that the BREC will need an especially significant budget, anticipating that—at least initially—it will principally serve a convening function with a modest staff, and that the remainder of its budget will otherwise go to circumscribed tasks such as data collection and analysis.

The participants in the BREC would be drawn from a diverse set of organizations and entities, including associations of academic institutions, federal agencies, industry groups, and not-for-profit organizations, including those that represent postdoctoral fellows and graduate students and those that advocate for the research enterprise. Membership can be set initially by an ad hoc sponsoring group consisting of the above stakeholder organizations, after which the BREC could choose its own members. The committee envisions that initially the BREC would be relatively modest in size, in the vicinity of 10 to 20 members. This number is small enough to allow for collaboration and effective deliberation, but large enough to represent the full scope of the biomedical research enterprise.

Long-Term BREC Structure

After the BREC is established and functional, it should transition to a self-supporting model of funding. One option is a tiered fee schedule that varies based on the type (profit, nonprofit, university, government agency) and size of institution (annual revenue or operating budget), to ensure that all relevant stakeholders can participate. Here too, precedents can be found in existing multi-stakeholder bodies.[7] The committee cannot predict with absolute certainty that stakeholders will provide the entirety of the financial support necessary to fund the BREC once it transitions away from exclusive NIH funding. But we are encouraged by the precedents whereby a membership fee, either alone or combined with other funding sources, has been successful in supporting multi-stakeholder public-private bodies in other arenas.

The committee considered alternatives to the creation of the BREC, such as remitting responsibility for the work to one of several existing scientific advisory bodies, such as the President's Council of Advisors on Science and Technology, but found that those bodies tend to be structured principally to provide counsel to the government on the development of its own science

---

[6] See https://www.gridwiseac.org/about/mission.aspx (accessed February 9, 2018).

[7] An example is the Smart Grid Interoperability Panel. Although this body includes a committee that is formed from larger plenary bodies, the membership fee is applied to the full plenary membership. (The Committee notes that a large plenary would not be incompatible with the concept of the BREC.)

policies, which is a very different role from that intended for the BREC. The committee also canvassed alternative options for the structure of the BREC that involve less formality or less robust representation and funding, but ultimately concluded that the need for sustained, legitimate oversight and coordination for a sector that is so critical to the nation's social and economic welfare required the establishment of this organization. To do less would render the effort susceptible to criticism by excluded stakeholders. The numerous related committee and task force reports over the years on the biomedical workforce (see Appendix B) underscore the desirability of a more streamlined and formal institution. An assessment of the utility and effectiveness of the BREC should be conducted 5 years after its establishment.

The committee envisions that the BREC would serve as a policy forum for conceptualizing and developing ideas focused on supporting early-career researchers, sharing information, convening workshops to assess progress, and evaluating and creating accountability for implementation of policy reforms. The BREC would anticipate future trends and needs in relation to challenges and opportunities confronting early-stage and early established investigators (ESIs and EEIs[8]) and would examine the extent to which research institutions and the private sector are creating adequate opportunities for early-career researchers to thrive. The BREC could play an early role in data collection (see Recommendations 3.3 and 3.4), an area with meaningful and encouraging momentum but relatively little interaction between public and private groups on what should be collected and how. The BREC should also examine the extent to which federal programs and policies—including recommended new policies and programs from this report that are implemented by NIH—are having their intended effects to support the next generation of biomedical researchers. Therefore, the committee makes the following recommendation:

Recommendation 3.1
Congress should establish a Biomedical Research Enterprise Council (BREC) to address ongoing challenges confronting the Next Generation of Biomedical Researchers. The BREC would exercise ongoing collective guardianship of the biomedical enterprise and function as a forum for sustained coordination, consultation, problem-solving, and assessment of progress toward implementation of the recommendations put forth in this report.

INCREASING DIVERSITY AND INCLUSION

One charge to the BREC would be to address the twin issues of disparity and inclusion. As described in Chapter 2, underrepresented minorities and women

---

[8] EEI is defined as "a Program Director/Principal Investigator (PD/PI) who is within 10 years of receiving their first substantial, independent competing NIH R01 equivalent research award as an ESI." https://grants.nih.gov/policy/early-investigators/index.htm (accessed February 15, 2018).

face enduring barriers to success, and the entire biomedical research enterprise must share responsibility for breaking down the barriers that prevent these populations from thriving and advancing in their chosen career paths. The capacity of the system to support the best science will be subverted if systemic barriers continue to thwart the recruitment of the brightest scientists irrespective of their race, gender, socioeconomic, or ethnic background.

There is little consensus on the effectiveness of potential strategies for improving diversity in the biomedical sciences. Few studies have evaluated or tested the impact of these strategies on the diversity or climate of institutions, and no studies that the committee could find assessed interventions in a systematic way across different institutional contexts. Notably, NIH has undertaken an extensive and ongoing review of its practices to improve diversity of the biomedical workforce. As a result of that review, NIH created the Scientific Workforce Diversity Office and the Diversity Program Consortium, the latter of which consists of three integrated initiatives—Building Infrastructure Leading to Diversity (BUILD), the National Research Mentoring Network (NRMN), and the Coordination and Evaluation Center (CEC). The CEC pilots and conducts rigorous evaluation and assessment of possible intervention strategies.

These programs, however, are supported by the NIH Common Fund, and are therefore not slated for funding after 10 years of operation. If the evaluations of these programs are positive, the nation's universities, research institutions, and government laboratories should draw on the findings to enhance their own diversity and inclusion initiatives in the biomedical arena. There is, in fact, growing evidence that institutional interventions aimed at enhancing workforce diversity can be effective. For instance, progress has been made in the development of strategies to increase gender representation among institutions participating in the NSF-ADVANCE program and of underrepresented populations in the National Institute of General Medical Sciences (NIGMS) Institutional Research and Academic Career Development Award (IRACDA) (K12) program. The IRACDA program, for example, funds postdoctoral training programs that combine a mentored research experience with an opportunity to develop additional academic and teaching skills. Currently, only 25 institutions have IRACDA programs, each supporting five to six postdoctoral researchers per year. A recent evaluation of the IRACDA program shows promising recruitment of underrepresented populations into the program, as well as a high rate of transition into academic careers compared to those postdoctoral researchers supported by Ruth L. Kirschstein National Research Service Award (NRSA) Individual Postdoctoral Fellowships (F32 award) over the same period (Faupel-Badger and Miklos, 2016).

Although NIH's continuing commitment to enhancing the diversity of the biomedical research enterprise is laudable, it is not, nor should it be, the only stakeholder championing adoption of these effective programs. Universities are well-positioned to identify evidence-based practices for their institutions and to implement and scale those practices on their own, in parallel with NIH's efforts to develop evidence-based reform. Through their training, educational, mentoring, and coaching programs, the biopharmaceutical industry and health care accelerators and incubators are also committed to increasing the participation of underrepresented populations and women in their research workforce. Accordingly, the committee makes the following recommendation to strengthen the excellence and diversity of the biomedical research enterprise:

Recommendation 3.2
All stakeholders in the biomedical research enterprise—universities, research institutions, government laboratories, and biomedical industries—should promote, document, assess, and disseminate their existing and planned efforts to reduce the barriers to recruiting and retaining diverse researchers at all stages of career development.

INCREASING TRANSPARENCY

The community's responses to the Dear Colleague Letter (see Appendix C) revealed widespread concern about the paucity of accurate, timely data to guide decision-making by and about the biomedical workforce, a concern that previous reports have also raised. As Chapter 2 details, the time and investment committed to building a career in biomedical research is substantial, yet, too often, trainees lack the information needed to make informed choices about career and training opportunities that align with their interests and talents. This absence of information also likely contributes to disequilibrium in the workforce characterized by a mismatch between the career aspirations of trainees and the jobs available in specific sectors of the biomedical research enterprise, particularly tenure-track faculty positions (Sauermann and Roach, 2012), and it reduces the potential positive impact of the federal government's—and hence taxpayers'—investment in training biomedical researchers.

There has been some promising recent activity with respect to collecting information to guide graduate student career choices. For example, the NIH Broadening Experiences in Scientific Training (BEST) consortium requires its members to collect and disseminate information on graduate student career outcomes. Universities such as Stanford University and Vanderbilt have been early leaders, and, on September 20, 2017, the Association of American Universities (AAU) issued a policy statement calling on "all Ph.D. granting universities and their respective Ph.D. granting colleges, schools and departments, to make a commitment to providing prospective and current students with easily accessible information."[9] The AAU statement stated explicitly that such data should include student demographics, average time to finish a degree, financial support, and career paths and outcomes both inside and outside academia.

---

[9] See https://www.insidehighered.com/quicktakes/2017/09/20/aau-sets-expectation-data-transparency-Ph.D.-program-outcomes (accessed November 22, 2017).

Other groups, such as Rescuing Biomedical Research[10] (RBR), the Council of Graduate Schools (CGS), and the newly formed Coalition for Next Generation Life Sciences (CNGLS) (Blank et al., 2017), are also mobilizing universities to improve transparency about Ph.D. career outcomes. RBR has worked with AAU, the Association of American Medical Colleges (AAMC), NIH, the BEST consortium, and numerous universities and other research organizations to develop a common set of methods for data collection on Ph.D. alumni and a common career outcomes taxonomy (Pickett and Tilghman, 2017). In October 2016, CGS announced a pilot program that will fund 15 universities to gather and use data about the careers of Ph.D. students and alumni in the humanities to support career development and mentoring,[11] and the Graduate Career Consortium has developed its own taxonomy for tracking Ph.D. career outcomes (Brinkman et al., 2017). In December 2017, CNGLS announced an agreement between its nine member universities and one research institution on a set of milestones for the next 2 years for collecting data on training outcomes for doctoral students and postdoctoral fellows, among other commitments. The presidents and chancellors of these universities acknowledged that "the arguments in favor of transparency are sound, and the time has come for institutions to develop credible mechanisms that are responsive to these concerns" (Blank et al., 2017, p. 1389).

The efforts mentioned above create an opportunity to guide the development of a multi-stakeholder plan for data transparency across research institutions and to ensure that data collection is consistent across universities and useful to trainees and policymakers alike. Given that universities are required to collect much of this information on trainees funded through NIH Ruth L. Kirschstein NRSA Institutional Research Training Grants (T32 award), and occasionally when hosting privately funded fellowships, the rationale for declining to share these data with prospective students is weak. Some institutions are not collecting and publishing such data because they fear that the necessary cost and time to do so would be prohibitive or that publication of career outcomes data would negatively affect their recruitment efforts, but the RBR effort found those fears to be unfounded. In fact, as the authors of a report on the RBR effort noted, "Interviews of institutions that had collected and published data on their biomedical Ph.D. alumni suggested that many of these roadblocks could be overcome with efficient data collection and presentation programs, and that their commitment to transparency actually enhanced graduate student recruiting rather than diminishing it" (Pickett and Tilghman, 2017, p.3).

Previous reports have called on research institutions to collect information on training outcomes and to make that information easily accessible for their students and postdoctoral trainees, yet most institutions have been slow to respond to these recommendations. The committee is encouraged that the many efforts on-

---

[10] See http://rescuingbiomedicalresearch.org/about/ (accessed December 8, 2017).

[11] See http://cgsnet.org/cgs-announces-multi-university-project-collect-data-career-pathways-humanities-Ph.D.s (accessed November 22, 2017).

going today to develop taxonomies for collecting data on educational and career outcomes for Ph.D. students will prompt the biomedical research community to join the burgeoning movement to increase transparency. Although it would be ideal for the community to reach consensus on one taxonomy, it is beyond the remit of this committee to recommend one taxonomy over another. At a minimum, though, the data collected should include Ph.D. completion rates, time to degree, length of time between attaining a Ph.D. and accepting an independent position, number and length of postdoctoral positions, and sector and location of employment for a minimum of 10 years after receiving the Ph.D., disaggregated to the extent possible by demographics, including gender, race and ethnicity, and visa status. Institutions should update these data on a regular schedule. Some research institutions have begun to clarify and narrow the number of titles and career tracks for postdoctoral researchers, which enable better collection on their status and outcomes, and other institutions should emulate this trend.

In addition to being invaluable to our young scientists, these data are critical for sound policymaking. For example, there is a debate in the literature about whether the asymmetries that exist in the biomedical workforce justify more draconian interventions, such as limits on graduate enrollments (Alberts et al., 2014; Stephan, 2012). The case in favor of such caps is based in no small measure on the increasing number of postdoctoral trainees relative to the number of available academic positions and the large and growing number of individuals with biomedical doctorates working in non-research positions. However, before taking a step as dramatic as reducing the number of students admitted to biomedical Ph.D. programs, it is crucial to understand the actual population of trainees, the duration of postdoctoral training, career trajectories and aspirations of trainees, changes in these data over time, and the type of research versus non-research positions that Ph.D.'s ultimately secure, including data on whether these placements are in the United States or abroad. Furthermore, if trainees were given the agency to make informed career choices using robust and timely information, their actions might contribute to balancing the supply and demand.

The committee makes the following two recommendations to address the need for increased transparency and data generation to support better private decisions and better policy development.

Recommendation 3.3
Biomedical research institutions should collect, analyze, and disseminate comprehensive data on outcomes, demographics, and career aspirations of biomedical pre- and postdoctoral researchers using common standards and definitions as developed by the institutions in concert with the National Institutes of Health (NIH). To incentivize compliance, NIH should make collection and publication of these data a requirement for additional NIH funding. This requirement should be phased-in over a 5-year period.

Recommendation 3.4
The National Science Foundation (NSF) should develop and implement a plan to improve sector-wide data collection and analysis in a manner that is easily accessible by policymakers and integrates data from numerous other sources. NSF should expeditiously link the Survey of Doctorate Recipients and the Survey of Earned Doctorates to U.S. Census data, and those linked data, under strict confidentiality protocols, should be made available for qualified researchers to use at Federal Statistical Research Data Centers to better understand the biomedical workforce.

NSF stands as the national clearinghouse of information collected through various surveys on science and engineering trainees and the workforce (see Box 3-1). Therefore, the committee recommends that NSF, which has developed an extensive infrastructure to collect these data, lead a renewed effort to improve the collection of sector-wide biomedical data, with an emphasis on standardizing, collecting, and synthesizing data from across the workforce. Currently, NIH contributes funds to support NSF's Survey of Doctoral Recipients and Survey of Earned Doctorates.

Additional efforts to synthesize data would benefit from the empirical infrastructure built since 2015 by the Institute for Research on Innovation and Science (IRIS), which provides a platform for linking university administrative records with U.S. Census data, as well as administrative data with other databases, including patents and publications.[12] Among the early insights into the careers of researchers produced using IRIS data is a better understanding of the factors contributing to an aging science and engineering workforce (Blau and Weinberg, 2017) and the geographic locations and sectors employing recent science and engineering Ph.D.'s (Zolas et al., 2015). Given the promising nature of the IRIS system, the committee strongly urges that research institutions join the IRIS initiative. This system is consistent and aligned with recommendations made by the Commission on Evidence-Based Policy Making (Commission on Evidence-Based Policymaking, 2017).

There have been multiple efforts recently to collect data about portions of the workforce, and the NIH Office of Extramural Programs (OER) has played a leadership role in such efforts. The committee appreciates the analytical support that it received from OER during its deliberations. In 2015, NIH established the Division of Biomedical Research Workforce Programs (DBRW)[13] within OER in part to analyze biomedical research workforce data. However, these data are not comprehensive; NIH is largely limited to information about its own grant programs, and broader data about the workforce are neither comprehensive, precise, nor readily available.

NIH funded the University of Minnesota to develop IPUMS Higher Ed,[14] a publicly available tool released in 2016 that harmonizes multiple NSF datasets—

---

[12] See http://iris.isr.umich.edu/ (accessed November 22, 2017).
[13] See https://researchtraining.nih.gov/dbrw (accessed November 22, 2017).
[14] See https://highered.ipums.org/highered/ (accessed November 22, 2017).

> **BOX 3-1**
> **NSF Data Surveys**
>
> - **National Survey of College Graduates** is a longitudinal biennial survey conducted since the 1970s that provides data on the nation's college graduates, with a focus on those in the science and engineering workforce. The survey samples individuals who are living in the United States during the survey reference period, have at least a bachelor's degree, and are under age 76. This survey is a unique source for examining the relationship of degree field and occupation in addition to other characteristics of college-educated individuals, including occupation, work activities, salary, and demographic information.
> - **The Survey of Doctorate Recipients (SDR)** provides demographic, education, and career history information for individuals with a U.S. research doctoral degree in a science, engineering, or health field. Conducted since 1973, the SDR is a unique source of information about the educational and occupational achievements and career movement of U.S.-trained doctoral scientists and engineers in the United States and abroad.
> - **The Survey of Earned Doctorates (SED)** is an annual census conducted since 1957 of all individuals receiving a research doctorate from an accredited U.S. institution in a given academic year. The SED collects information on the doctoral recipient's educational history, demographic characteristics, and postgraduation plans. Results are used to assess characteristics of the doctoral population and trends in doctoral education and degrees.
> - **The Graduate Students and Postdoctorates in Science and Engineering Survey** is an annual census of all U.S. academic institutions granting research-based master's degrees or doctorates in science, engineering, and selected health fields as of fall of the survey year. The survey collects the total number of graduate students, postdoctoral appointees, and doctorate-level non-faculty researchers by demographic and other characteristics such as source of financial support. Results are used to assess shifts in graduate enrollment and postdoctoral appointments and trends in financial support.
> - **Science and Engineering Indicators,** compiled by NSF, under guidance of the National Science Board, and delivered to Congress and the President by January 15 each even numbered year, are quantitative representations relevant to the scope, quality, and vitality of the science and engineering enterprise. The report is a factual and policy-neutral source of high-quality U.S. and international data that contributes to the understanding of the U.S. science and engineering enterprise within a global context.

the National and International Survey of Doctoral Recipients (SDR) databases and Survey of College Graduates (NSCG) and National Survey of Recent College Graduates (NSRCG) databases—from 1990 to 2013. IPUMS Higher Ed provides a user-friendly data extraction system to track career trajectories of Ph.D.'s across different occupations, including in academia, government, industry, and research organizations. These actions represent an important first step toward addressing the information gap, but they are limited by inconsistent institutional data collection efforts and a lack of transparency.

SUSTAINABILITY

Unpredictable biomedical research funding impairs long-term planning and reverberates across a workforce that relies on stable financial support and highly trained researchers. As noted in Chapter 2, the decline in real dollars of federal research support has contributed directly to the many stresses facing the incoming generation of biomedical researchers. For example, ESIs securing their first NIH award must deal with the declining purchasing power of those awards. Over the past decade, the size of grant awards has not tracked with research inflation as measured by the Biomedical Research and Development Price Index calculated by the Bureau of Economic Analysis. Today, investigators must fund their research with an award that is worth approximately 80 percent of its value 10 years ago.[15] The decline in funding in constant dollars, and the resulting sharp increase in competition for the available funding, has also meant that NIH has had fewer opportunities to address enduring barriers to groundbreaking research for the next generation of biomedical researchers.

Over the years, a series of thoughtful and evidence-based reports from a cadre of leaders in biomedical research have called for solutions. Many of these solutions have been reiterated in report after report, including doubling the number of Pathway to Independence (K99/R00) awards and the NIH Director's Early Independence Awards (DP5), with the goal of easing the transition of trainees to independent research positions, increasing the proportion of postdoctoral researchers supported by training grants and fellowships, and developing new programs for early faculty that seek to respond to particular barriers they face in developing new research programs (FASEB, 2015; Institute of Medicine et al., 2000; National Academy of Sciences et al., 2014; National Research Council, 2005). However, as highlighted in Appendix B, NIH has not fully implemented these recommendations.

In addition, unpredictable funding or periodic surges and subsequent cuts in the NIH budget create issues for a research enterprise that depends on long-term planning and multi-year grants. These issues can place a unique burden on early-career investigators, who are especially vulnerable to unpredictable funding for NIH. More importantly, the United States is in danger of squandering its global competitive edge in biomedical research as other nations build their research investments and create incentives to recruit their research talent back from our training programs and laboratories and as the United States grapples with various immigration issues that affect the ability of biomedical researchers

---

[15] See https://officeofbudget.od.nih.gov/pdfs/FY18/BRDPI%20Table%20FY%201950%20to%202022_Jan%202017.pdf (accessed December 5, 2017).

with temporary visa holders to remain in this country (National Science Board, 2018). For these reasons, a wide range of respected organizations in recent years, including the National Academies (National Academy of Sciences et al., 2007; National Research Council, 2012), the American Academy of Arts & Sciences (2014), and United for Medical Research (2015) have called for more dependable funding for basic research.

In August 2017, NIH launched the Next Generation Researchers Initiative (NGRI) specifically to provide additional funding for ESIs and EEIs to "promote the growth, stability and diversity of the biomedical research workforce."[16] NIH Director Francis Collins explained in a June 8, 2017, letter that the funding required to carry out this policy would be drawn from commitments already made in the 2017 NIH base budget, and then, pending the availability of funds, investment in the initiative would increase to $1.1 billion per year after 5 years. Although the NGRI could address many of the funding challenges unique to ESIs and EEIs, its current structure requires NIH to support it with funds currently allocated to other initiatives and research needs. This would divert funds from more established investigators and would increase the hyper-competition for funding, threatening the sustainability of the enterprise and decreasing the amount of funds available for these researchers when they no longer qualify for an award under the NGRI.

Therefore, to fully realize the promise of initiatives aimed at helping the next generation of biomedical researchers, including the NGRI and the recommendations in this report, Congress should provide new funds for their implementation in the same manner it has for initiatives such as the Human Genome Project, the Cancer Genome Atlas Project, the Brain Research through Advancing Innovative Neurotechnologies (BRAIN) Initiative, and the NIH *All of Us* Research Study. To ensure consistent funding for the incoming generations of independent investigators and the vibrancy of the biomedical research enterprise and its workforce, Congress should increase its annual funding for NIH at a rate that is at least equal to the Biomedical Research and Development Price Index developed by the Bureau of Economic Analysis.

As noted throughout this report, evidence shows that securing federal research funding, particularly R01 support, has become increasingly competitive over the past decade. At the same time, because increases in federal support for NIH have been modest, the purchasing power of NIH grants have diminished over that period. This heightened competition affects all researchers, but especially early-career scientists without a strong record of grant success.

The Statement of Task for this study explicitly requires the committee to analyze the full range of barriers and constraints to research opportunities for career researchers. It reads, in part, "The study will include . . . an evaluation of the impact of federal policies and budgets. . . ." Any serious effort to address the barriers faced by early-career scientists cannot ignore the challenges of reduced funding

---

[16] See https://grants.nih.gov/ngri.htm (accessed December 15, 2017).

and more intense competition for scarce research dollars—to say nothing of the challenges presented by the lack of predictable, sustained funding that arises as a result of annual uncertainties in the Congressional appropriations process.

As such, the committee includes a recommendation not only for support of new and enhanced programmatic initiatives at NIH, and more aggressive policies and programs at research institutions, but also for an increase in overall Congressional appropriations for NIH to support the NGRI and enable expansion of programs, such as the NIH BEST program, that address some of the early biomedical career issues discussed in this report. The committee is not proposing sweeping programs that require substantial money. Indeed, the financial scale of its recommendations, estimated to cost approximately $1 billion over 5 years, is small relative to that of research project grant funding, yet such funds would substantially increase resources available for training, mentoring, and sustaining the careers of ESIs.

If Congress provides no additional funding for NIH, and funds cannot be reallocated within the agency, then many of the trends discussed throughout this report (e.g., increasing age to securing an R01-equivalent grant, decreasing representation of NIH-supported investigators under age 50, enduring barriers to diversifying the research workforce, and prevailing lack of accountability for the training and mentorship of postdoctoral researchers) may very well continue, or even worsen. If Congress provides no additional funding and NIH reallocates funds from research grants, then these problems could continue and even pose additional challenges when investigators try to secure subsequent NIH funding. As discussed throughout this report, additional considerations influence the trajectory of the biomedical workforce independent of funding. However, in the years since the 2005 *Bridges to Independence* report, congressional funding for NIH research has declined in real dollars, and although NIH has sought to commit funding and attention to address the challenges facing young investigators, a number of the recommendations were not fully implemented, and the problems have endured.

A commitment of funding is necessary to bend the curve on these issues and to achieve the vision of a truly dynamic and innovative workforce system. Otherwise, we seem destined to repeat the lessons of the past. Therefore, the committee recommends the following:

Recommendation 3.5
Congress should consider increasing the National Institutes of Health (NIH) budget specifically to support implementation of the recommendations in this report and to provide sustained support for NIH's recently announced Next Generation Researchers Initiative.

REFERENCES

Alberts, B., M. W. Kirschner, S. Tilghman, and H. Varmus. 2014. Rescuing US biomedical research from its systemic flaws. *Proceedings of the National Academy of Sciences of the United States of America* 111(16):5773-5777.

American Academy of Arts and Sciences. 2014. *Restoring the foundation: The vital role of research in preserving the American dream.* Cambridge, MA: American Academy of Arts and Sciences.

Blank, R., R. J. Daniels, G. Gilliland, A. Gutmann, S. Hawgood, F. A. Hrabowski, M. E. Pollack, V. Price, L. R. Reif, and M. S. Schlissel. 2017. A new data effort to inform career choices in biomedicine. *Science* 358(6369):1388-1389.

Blau, D. M., and B. A. Weinberg. 2017. Why the US science and engineering workforce is aging rapidly. *Proceedings of the National Academy of Sciences* 114(15):3879-3884.

Brinkman, J., J. Locher, A. Bankston, S. Gadwal, M. Sinche, and H. Morgan. 2017. Trends in PhD careers outcomes tracking. *F1000Research* 6:1022 (poster). https://f1000research.com/posters/6-1022 (accessed February 7, 2018).

Commission on Evidence-Based Policymaking. 2017. *The promise of evidence-based policymaking.* Washington, DC: U.S. Government Printing Office.

Daniels, R. 2015. A generation at risk: Young investigators and the future of the biomedical workforce. *Proceedings of the National Academy of Sciences of the United States of America* 112(2): 313-318.

FASEB (Federation for American Societies for Experimental Biology). 2015. *Sustaining discovery in biological and medical sciences: A framework for discussion.* Bethesda, MD: Federation of American Societies for Experimental Biology.

Faupel-Badger, J., and A. Miklos. 2016. *Institutional Research and Academic Career Development Awards (IRACDA) (K12) outcomes assessment.* Bethesda, MD: National Institute of General Medical Sciences.

Institute of Medicine, National Academy of Sciences, and National Academy of Engineering. 2000. *Enhancing the postdoctoral experience for scientists and engineers: A guide for postdoctoral scholars, advisers, institutions, funding organizations, and disciplinary societies.* Washington, DC: The National Academies Press.

National Academy of Sciences, National Academy of Engineering, and Institute of Medicine. 2007. *Rising above the gathering storm: Energizing and employing America for a brighter economic future.* Washington, DC: The National Academies Press.

National Academy of Sciences, National Academy of Engineering, and Institute of Medicine. 2014. *The postdoctoral experience revisited.* Washington, DC: The National Academies Press.

National Research Council. 2005. *Bridges to independence: Fostering the independence of new investigators in biomedical research.* Washington, DC: The National Academies Press.

National Research Council. 2012. *Research universities and the future of America: Ten breakthrough actions vital to our nation's prosperity and security.* Washington, DC: The National Academies Press.

National Science Board. 2018. *Science and engineering indicators 2018.* Alexandria, VA: National Science Foundation.

Pickett, C. L., and S. Tilghman. 2017. Becoming more transparent: Collecting and presenting data on biomedical Ph.D. alumni. *PeerJ Preprints* 5:e3370v1, https://doi.org/10.7287/peerj.preprints.3370v1 (accessed February 6, 2018).

Sauermann, H., and M. Roach. 2012. Science PhD career preferences: Levels, changes, and advisor encouragement. *PloS One* 7(5):e36307.

Stephan, P. E. 2012. *How economics shapes science.* Cambridge, MA: Harvard University Press.

United for Medical Research. 2015. Healthy Funding: Ensuring a Predictable and Growing Budget for the National Institutes of Health, http://www.unitedformedicalresearch.com/wp-content/uploads/2015/02/2_18-UMR-Final-copy.pdf (accessed March 14, 2018).

Zolas, N., N. Goldschlag, R. Jarmin, P. Stephan, J. Owen-Smith, R. F. Rosen, B. M. Allen, B. A. Weinberg, and J. I. Lane. 2015. Wrapping it up in a person: Examining employment and earnings outcomes for Ph.D. recipients. *Science* 350(6266):1367-1371.

4

Transitioning to Independence

The federal government makes a substantial investment in future scientists through a variety of training and research grant mechanisms. These individuals make their own investment, by devoting upwards of 12 years of time, intellect, and skills to prepare for a career in biomedical research after obtaining a bachelor's degree.[1] Considering the magnitude of this public and private investment, it is imperative that they receive comprehensive and meaningful research training, mentorship, and, as discussed in Chapter 3, the information needed to find and then thrive in a career that aligns with their interests and talents. This is essential for the United States to retain its leadership role in biomedical research and advancements.

As of 2013, 80 percent of U.S. biomedical Ph.D.'s enter postdoctoral research training after receiving their doctoral degrees (Kahn and Ginther, 2017). Most individuals enter into a postdoctoral research position with the intention of becoming an academic research faculty member (Sauermann and Roach, 2012), but only 18 percent ultimately secure tenure-track or tenured positions within 10 years of obtaining their doctorates (Figure 2-1). Others enter postdoctoral training to prepare for industry or other non-academic positions, while others do not state any clear career goal (Gibbs et al., 2015).

As explained in Chapter 2, the postdoctoral experience should be a mentored transition to research independence with the purpose of providing additional scientific, technical, and professional skills to advance an individual's career. However, as also explained in Chapter 2, postdoctoral researchers have long been

---

[1] In this report, "biomedical" refers to the full range of biological, biomedical, behavioral, and health sciences supported by the National Institutes of Health.

recognized as valuable to the research enterprise, "performing a substantial portion of the nation's research in every setting" (Institute of Medicine et al., 2000, p. 10). The tension between the roles of trainee and institutional employee can taint the postdoctoral experience and compromise opportunities for postdoctoral researchers to develop the skills needed for their eventual careers. Trainee status, for example, typically entails low wages relative to the postdoctoral researcher's educational background, and studies indicate that it can take up to 15 years after degree attainment for the postdoctoral cohort to catch up in salary compared to the non-postdoctoral cohort. To the extent that trainees are forgoing higher wages[2] and benefits for a limited time period in exchange for meaningful opportunities to advance their long-term career goals, this trade-off is not controversial. However, if trainees are languishing in low-paying jobs, not securing appropriate mentorship and training, not progressing steadily toward research independence, and not receiving counseling about other potential career tracks (i.e., as a staff scientist), the situation becomes deeply problematic and violates core academic norms and values.

Although biomedical researchers throughout the enterprise face a variety of challenges during their research careers,[3] the challenges experienced during the postdoctoral research stage command explicit attention in this report (Gibbs et al., 2015; Institute of Medicine et al., 2000; Kahn and Ginther, 2017; National Academy of Sciences et al., 2014). To address these issues, the committee makes the following set of recommendations.

TRAINING AND SUPPORT FOR ALL POSTDOCTORAL RESEARCHERS

Recommendation 4.1

Research institutions, principal investigators (PIs), and federal funding agencies should each play their part to support transitions from Ph.D.'s, M.D.'s, and M.D.-Ph.D.'s. to research independence by providing every postdoctoral researcher, regardless of the support mechanism or training location, with a high-quality training experience that prepares them for success in their chosen career. To achieve this overarching objective:

- **The National Institutes of Health (NIH) should require the inclusion of an institutional training and mentoring plan as a component of**

---

[2] National Science Board. Science & Engineering Indicators 2018, Table 3-18: Median salaries for recent U.S. SEH doctorate recipients in postdoc and non-postdoc positions up to 5 years after receiving degree: 2015. https://www.nsf.gov/statistics/2018/nsb20181/assets/901/tables/tt03-18.pdf (accessed February 28, 2018).

[3] The National Academies' Committee on Revitalizing Graduate STEM Education is addressing these same issues from the perspective of graduate training in science, technology, engineering, and mathematics.

the "Resources and Environment" reported on research and training grant applications. In addition, NIH should require PIs to provide a postdoctoral research training and mentoring plan in all grant proposals, as well as updates on those plans in annual and interim research performance progress reports for funded proposals.
- **Research institutions should provide evidence to NIH of formal training of faculty mentors of postdoctoral trainees.**
- **Research institutions should introduce a mechanism to facilitate career guidance counseling for all postdoctoral researchers. This mechanism would preferably begin in the first year but must occur no later than the third year of postdoctoral training. Such guidance should assess the postdoctoral researchers' progress and evaluate alignment of their career aspirations with career prospects.**
- **NIH should increase the Ruth L. Kirschstein National Research Service Award (NRSA) starting salary for new postdoctoral researchers to $52,700 (in 2018 dollars), with annual adjustments for inflation and for cost-of-living increases tied to the Personal Consumption Expenditure Index. Research institutions should adjust their base postdoctoral salary annually to match the corresponding NRSA rate, with adjustments based on local cost-of-living, and they should harmonize benefits for all postdoctoral scholars regardless of support mechanism.**
- **Research institutions should levy a fee of at least $1,000 per year, to be paid by the host investigator, for each postdoctoral fellow on all biomedical research grants. Funds from the fee would be used to support effective training and professional development programs for postdoctoral researchers, as well as effective training of mentors. Research institutions should report publicly on the use of the money generated by this fee.**
- **All research institutions should, following best practices, identify or provide an institutional ombudsperson to resolve fairly and expeditiously conflicts and concerns between PIs and postdoctoral researchers related to training experiences.**

For the purposes of this report, "postdoctoral researchers" are advanced trainees who, by definition, are entitled to receive training and mentoring regardless of the funding mechanism that supports them. This approach aligns with recommendations made by NIH, the American Association of Medical Colleges (AAMC), the National Postdoctoral Association (NPA), and the Office of Management and Budget (OMB).[4]

---

[4] See Box 2-1 and NIH Notice NOT-OD-15-008, https://grants.nih.gov/grants/guide/notice-files/NOT-OD-15-008.html (accessed February 8, 2018).

Currently, approximately 46 percent of biomedical postdoctoral researchers at universities are supported on research project grants (RPGs).[5] Unlike training grants and individual fellowships, RPGs do not *explicitly* require postdoctoral training or career development activities or reports on training outcomes. Further, the peer review process for RPGs focuses on the merit of the proposed project and does not assess the PI's training record or the quality of the experiences of postdoctoral researchers supported on the grant. Postdoctoral researchers supported on RPGs during their entire tenure lack external benchmarks (such as the need to develop their own research project for a fellowship application) that could encourage and recognize the development of research independence. In addition, RPGs are awarded to PIs and therefore are not portable by postdoctoral researchers, making them dependent upon the PI for salary and research support. Finally, the use of RPG funding for postdoctoral researchers makes it more difficult to monitor the number of postdoctoral researchers and to assess their career progress.

Even if the number of fellowships and training grants were to be increased substantially as recommended below, postdoctoral researchers will remain supported largely through RPGs for the near future, given that only 10 percent of postdoctoral researchers are currently supported on federal fellowships and traineeships.[6] Nonetheless, select changes in the RPG application and peer review could hold both the PI and the institution accountable for postdoctoral research training and thereby reduce disparities between training experiences. To start, NIH should require that the "Resources and Environment" section in all grant applications includes an institutional training and mentoring plan, as well as an individualized plan that outlines the PI's commitment to the scientific and professional development of all postdoctoral research trainees. These additional requirements would build upon the existing requirement that NIH annual progress reports describe how individual development plans (IDPs) help to identify and promote the career goals of graduate students and postdoctoral researchers associated with NIH awards.[7] This recommendation encourages research institutions to take responsibility for developing robust training and mentoring programs for their postdoctoral researchers.

This recommendation also contemplates a new mechanism to facilitate consideration by the researcher and their mentors of the researcher's credible career opportunities, based on their demonstrated commitment to, and capacity for, rigorous, creative, and meaningful independent research activity. This career guidance mechanism should be documented and should occur between the first

---

[5] NIH Data Book. Primary Source of Support for Postdoctorates. https://report.nih.gov/NIHDatabook/Charts/Default.aspx?showm=Y&chartId=263&catId=20 (accessed December 14, 2017).

[6] NIH Data Book. Primary Source of Support for Postdoctorates. https://report.nih.gov/NIHDatabook/Charts/Default.aspx?showm=Y&chartId=263&catId=20 (accessed December 14, 2017).

[7] NIH Notice NOT-OD-14-113. https://grants.nih.gov/grants/guide/notice-files/NOT-OD-14-113.html (accessed February 8, 2018).

and third year of the RPG or postdoctoral fellowship support. The committee envisions that every postdoctoral researcher would receive a written career guidance report that is signed by the PI and researcher and co-signed by the departmental head/chair. A final report would be included in any RPG or fellowship proposal that requests continued funding for that postdoctoral researcher. Following that report, each postdoctoral researcher would propose a concrete career plan, such as an IDP. Those aspiring to an academic research career would be expected to apply for an F or K award to continue preparation for an independent research career. Those ending their postdoctoral training would receive a reasonable time period to secure other employment. The discussions about career opportunities should cover a diversity of career paths, because the majority of biomedical Ph.D.'s do not transition into academic research positions (National Institutes of Health, 2012).

The collection of a modest fee for each postdoctoral researcher would create a partial funding source for institutional programs, including those that enhance training activities that occur outside the research laboratory, and would provide postdoctoral trainees with the resources, skills, and knowledge needed to succeed within and outside of academe. The imposition of an explicit, transparent fee in the RPG also reinforces the mentorship and training responsibilities of PIs and their home institutions. The amount of $1,000 is not so large that it will disrupt the RPG budgets, but is large enough to not only contribute funds to institutional programs, but also make PIs more cognizant of non-salary costs to employ and train postdoctoral researchers and to consider these costs when deciding whether or not to hire a postdoctoral researcher.[8] For institutions employing fewer than 100 postdoctoral researchers, the sum raised will be relatively modest but sufficient to encourage them to augment programs to enhance the training and employability of their postdoctoral researchers. Federal funding agencies should make this fee an allowable and itemized direct cost budget item, and institutions should be accountable for and report the use of the fee.

Regarding the specific training that postdoctoral researchers should expect to receive, the committee endorses the six core competencies cited by the National Postdoctoral Association: (1) discipline-specific conceptual knowledge, (2) research skill development, (3) communication skills, (4) professionalism, (5) leadership and management skills, and (6) responsible conduct of research.[9] Peer review for grant proposals should evaluate both laboratory-based and institutional plans for trainees, adopting these competencies as criteria and rating as "ACCEPTABLE/UNACCEPTABLE," analogous to evaluations of the use of human subjects, the inclusion of children in research, and the use of vertebrate

---

[8] In economic terms, the tax reflects the cost of university-provided training that otherwise is exported from the lab to the university, thereby providing better information to PIs about the full cost of engaging a postdoctoral researcher in their labs.

[9] See http://www.nationalpostdoctoral researcher.org/page/CoreCompetencies (accessed November 24, 2017).

animals. Any concerns should be resolved before applications are recommended for funding.

Currently, stipends paid to postdoctoral researchers supported on RPGs are at the discretion of the PI. Although institutions establish guidelines, they may be optional or not enforced. *Postdoctoral Experience Revisited* (National Academy of Sciences et al., 2014) includes a recommendation that postdoctoral research salaries start at $50,000 in 2014 dollars. The committee considers this recommendation sound and endorses its adoption for all starting postdoctoral researchers. NIH has already revised NRSA stipend levels since the publication of this 2014 report, and many institutions base their postdoctoral research salary guidelines on these levels (National Academy of Sciences et al., 2014). Encouragingly, recent survey data show that institutions employing 60 percent of the U.S. postdoctoral population have instituted policies to raise postdoctoral salaries (Bankston and McDowell, 2017). The committee believes that this salary level should be adjusted periodically for inflation (meaning that the baseline salary would be $52,700 in 2018 dollars[10]) and for local cost-of-living increases (using existing federal guidelines). Institutions should also provide postdoctoral researchers with fringe benefits appropriate for advanced trainees as cited by the National Postdoctoral Association[11] and should make these benefits equitable across the institution, regardless of the source of postdoctoral research support.

The dependent status of most postdoctoral researchers—including a lack of job security, an inability to transfer salary support to a different laboratory, and the fact that their advisor will serve as a professional reference—renders them particularly vulnerable to instances of unfair or exploitative treatment. Therefore, each institution should appoint an ombudsperson to fairly and expeditiously resolve conflicts and concerns between PIs and postdoctoral researchers related to training experience, authorship disputes, and other matters. To be effective and credible, the office must be an impartial and independent actor and not saddled with responsibilities outside its narrow mandate (i.e., the broad employment and training issues relevant to postdoctoral researchers).

OPTIMIZING THE DURATION AND SUPPORT MECHANISMS FOR POSTDOCTORAL TRAINING

All postdoctoral researchers should be offered a mentored transition to independence and opportunities to develop skills and acquire substantive knowledge in their area of intended research. They should also be afforded opportunities to ascertain, in a timely manner and in concert with their mentors, suitable career trajectories following their postdoctoral experience. Given that the postdoctoral experience should be temporary, NIH, prior National Academies study commit-

---

[10] Bureau of Labor Statistics, CPI Calculator. https://data.bls.gov/cgi-bin/cpicalc.pl?cost1=50000&year1=201401&year2=201801 (accessed February 27, 2018).

[11] See http://www.nationalpostdoc.org/?recommpostdocpolicy (accessed December 15, 2017).

tees, research institutions, and scientific professional societies recommend limits on the length of postdoctoral training (see Appendix B).

Many argue that 5 years is an appropriate timeframe (see Appendix B) for postdoctoral researchers to complete training in preparation for an independent research career, while protecting them from languishing in a professional rank with little opportunity for career advancement. In the current climate, however, 5 years may not provide enough time for postdoctoral fellows to compete successfully for an academic research position. At the same time, 5 years is too long for timely consideration of other research and non-research career options. Although adopted by many universities, there has been little evidence that the 5-year rule on its own has substantially shortened the length of time spent in postdoctoral research positions, or has led to marked improvements in the training or mentoring experiences of postdoctoral researchers (Kahn and Ginther, 2017).

As discussed above and in Chapter 2, there are several respects in which RPGs present suboptimal training and mentoring support for postdoctoral researchers as compared to individual fellowships or mentored awards. Postdoctoral researchers on fellowships performed better on all outcomes compared to postdoctoral researchers on RPGs and training grants (National Institutes of Health, 2012). Indeed, it has been identified as potentially disadvantageous for underrepresented populations to be supported on RPGs rather than fellowship mechanisms (Working Group on Diversity in the Biomedical Research Workforce, 2012). Because PIs spend a large percentage of their time applying for funding, grantsmanship is a key skill for research independence in academia. Therefore, applying for an individual fellowship should become a standard practice during the postdoctoral training experience.

Thus, postdoctoral researchers would be better served if they secured their own support through individual awards that "diminish the employment relationship between postdoc and principal investigator" (National Research Council, 2005, p. 5). Although many PIs meaningfully train and mentor the postdoctoral researchers supported on their RPGs, it is challenging to guarantee these experiences for all postdoctoral researchers under an RPG where the primary accountable party is the PI.

In the public input received by this committee, a broad array of individuals and organizations shared the view that postdoctoral researchers should receive mentored training. As examples from the latter, the AAMC stated that "the research community should begin to disentangle 'workforce' from 'training'," and the Federation of American Societies for Experimental Biology recommended action to "help mitigate the current dualism that graduate students and postdoctoral researchers face as trainees AND employees." To address this persistent challenge, the committee recommends an approach to ease postdoctoral researchers off a funding mechanism that does not explicitly promote a mentored transition to an independent career, while also presenting a natural check-point, well before the 5-year mark, that motivates postdoctoral researchers and their advisers to actively consider the researcher's training and career trajectory.

Therefore, the committee recommends the following:

Recommendation 4.2
The National Institutes of Health (NIH) should expand existing awards or create new competitive awards to support postdoctoral researchers' advancement of their own independent research and to support professional development toward an independent research career. Both domestic and foreign postdoctoral researchers should be eligible for these awards. Over the next 5 years, NIH should incrementally and steadily increase by 5-fold the number of individual research fellowship awards (F-type) and career development (K-type) awards for postdoctoral researchers. The award recipients' home institutions should provide them with benefits commensurate to those provided to postdoctoral researchers supported on NIH research project grants and appropriate to their level of experience. The increase should not come at the expense of institutional training grants. The indirect cost recovery rate earned by K-type and training grant awards should be increased to 16 percent.

Recommendation 4.3
The National Institutes of Health (NIH) should phase in a cap (3 years suggested) on salary support for all postdoctoral researchers funded by NIH research project grants (RPGs) based on the following considerations:

- **The cap should not apply to time spent on fellowships or career development awards;**
- **The phase-in should occur only after NIH undertakes a robust pilot study (or studies) of sufficient size and duration to assess the feasibility of this policy and provide opportunities to revise it;**
- **The pilot study (or studies) should be coupled to action on recommendation 4.2, which calls for an increase in individual F and K awards that are not restricted to U.S. citizens and permanent residents;**
- **The pilot study (or studies) should assess potential benefits as well as potential deleterious consequences of such a cap for postdoctoral researchers, with special emphasis on women, underrepresented racial and ethnic minorities, and individuals with disabilities; early-stage independent investigators; and research creativity;**
- **A short extension of RPG support can be requested, with sufficient justification, to offset time lost because of unplanned circumstances (e.g., illness, lab disaster) or parental responsibilities; and**
- **Postdoctoral researchers should be allowed sufficient time between their last fellowship decision and the termination of their funding on RPGs to enable smooth career transitions.**

Recommendation 4.4
Postdoctoral training should be limited to 5 years, after which time any postdoctoral researcher continuing in the same laboratory should be shifted to employment as a staff scientist with an increase in salary and benefits as appropriate for a permanent staff member.

Recommendations 4.2, 4.3, and 4.4 are premised on the belief that limiting the time postdoctoral researchers are supported on an RPG rather than fellowship will diminish the risk that the researcher will linger in a research position without clear and meaningful opportunities for advancement, training, and mentorship.

Recommendation 4.2 seeks to address the concern that the current number of available fellowships is much smaller than the number of postdoctoral researchers, and it has declined in real terms over time even though previous reports have recommended its increase, as noted in Appendix B. Of postdoctoral researchers specifically supported by NIH in 2016, approximately 79 percent were supported on RPGs and 19 percent on a fellowship or traineeship.[12] To begin to shift the training system away from RPGs and toward a more beneficial platform for the next generation of researchers, the committee strongly advocates for a substantial increase in the proportion of postdoctoral researchers supported by F-type and K-type awards. These awards enable postdoctoral researchers to pursue research of their own design, and their portability ensures a suitable mentoring experience by tying the postdoctoral researchers to a project rather than a particular PI. Furthermore, peer review of F- and K-type applications ensures that postdoctoral fellows are selected for their potential to make significant scientific contributions rather than to serve as a productive subordinate.

The committee specifically recommends increases in independent F- and K-type awards rather than training grants. The committee considered various increases in F- and K-type awards, including a 10-fold increase. However, the committee concluded that a 5-fold increase in the number of F- and K-type awards over 5 years is preferable. Slightly more than 1,200 F-type awards[13] and nearly 1,000 K-type awards[14] were distributed in 2016, and a 5-fold increase would represent a substantial increase in the number of fellowships and career development awards and would help to transform the training landscape. These awards are not intended to increase the size of the postdoctoral researcher popula-

---

[12] NSF. Survey of Graduate Students and Postdoctorates in Science and Engineering, 2016, Table 41: Postdoctoral appointees in science, engineering, and health in all institutions, by field, primary source of support, and primary mechanism of support: 2016. https://ncsesdata.nsf.gov/gradpostdoc/2016/html/GSS2016_DST_41.html (accessed March 6, 2018).

[13] See https://report.nih.gov/NIHDatabook/Charts/Default.aspx?showm=Y&chartId=52&catId=17 (accessed February 9, 2018).

[14] See https://report.nih.gov/NIHDatabook/Charts/Default.aspx?showm=Y&chartId=211&catId=16 (accessed February 9, 2018).

tion, but instead to shift their support from RPGs, which are currently the most prevalent source of postdoctoral support.[15]

Prior recommendations for general increases in the numbers of postdoctoral researchers supported on fellowships (see Appendix B) have not gained traction. To the committee's knowledge, this recommendation is the first of this kind to set a concrete goal for such an increase. The committee recognizes the possibility that a large, non-staged increase could have unintended consequences for other aspects of the biomedical research enterprise, including the number and size of research grants, increased pressure on award reviewers, and the functioning and operation of laboratories. In particular, an expansion of F- and K-type awards might unintentionally penalize applications from postdoctoral researchers in the labs of early-stage investigators (ESIs) if they were deemed less competitive than those in the labs of established investigators.

The increase from 8 percent to 16 percent for indirect costs on F- and K-type awards is necessary to cover the incremental costs of multiple demands on training institutions to improve monitoring and reporting of the professional development and mentoring that trainees receive. Without a significant increase in the indirect costs associated with training grants, the new requirements outlined throughout this report would amount to an unfunded mandate and, as a result, would likely not be acted on in the manner needed.

Recommendation 4.3 creates an expectation that postdoctoral researchers who continue in positions supported by RPGs for more than a certain time period must transition to F- and K- awards (or similar awards from non-federal sources). This recommendation seeks to reinforce the decision point when the postdoctoral researcher and mentor should assess the researcher's potential to develop an independent research project. This decision point is not meant to determine a researcher's subsequent career choice; rather, it is meant to require the researcher to design and propose a fellowship project as a milestone on the path toward independence.

The committee suggests 3 years as an appropriate timeframe to support a postdoctoral fellow on an RPG, but recognizes that this timeframe should be examined in the pilot study (or studies). It is instructive that the authoring committee of *Bridges to Independence* expressed its hope that "the normal length of postdoctoral training will be closer to 3 years, whether in one or multiple environments. This is consistent with an overall training period—including graduate and postdoctoral training—of no more than 10 years" (National Research Council, 2005, p. 5). The committee recognizes, however, that in the current labor market, few postdoctoral researchers can compete for an independent position after only 3 years.

Therefore, postdoctoral researchers with strong potential to establish their own research programs (from all populations, including non-domestic, underrepresented ethnic and racial minorities, women, and individuals with disabili-

---

[15] NIH Data Book. Primary Source of Support for Postdoctorates. https://report.nih.gov/NIHDatabook/Charts/Default.aspx?showm=Y&chartId=263&catId=20 (accessed December 14, 2017).

ties) should continue their work on a funding mechanism that nurtures and promotes the development of their independence. For postdoctoral researchers who are phasing out after 3 years on an RPG, there must be an adequate number of opportunities for additional (but time-limited) support in the form of grants, fellowships, or awards that will allow them to complete their postdoctoral work and advance toward an independent academic research appointment—either in the United States or abroad.

The committee does not envision that the 3 years of support on research grants must run consecutively. One scenario for application of the cap could be 3 years of support on the PI's grant, and then a fellowship or career development award, but other scenarios are possible. The suggested 3-year cap should include a grace period of at least 1 year for parental leave to ensure that researchers with increasing family responsibilities are not selectively harmed by this policy change. The committee is mindful as well that the success of this recommendation depends on the application of a universal definition of a postdoctoral researcher, as noted in Chapter 2. Postdoctoral researchers who remain on a RPG for more than 3 years should be identified as a staff or career scientist and compensated accordingly.

The committee recognizes these recommended changes to current funding policies could have unpredictable effects on the incentives and conduct of researchers. Committee members had diverse and intensely held opinions about the likely impacts of implementing a 3-year cap on support from RPGs. In the end, committee members agreed that before any cap is instituted, NIH should develop one or more pilot studies to assess the feasibility of the recommendation and its consequences for research personnel across the biomedical research enterprise. These studies should begin expeditiously, be designed with sufficient size and duration for adequate assessment and evaluation, and be monitored by both NIH and the proposed Biomedical Research Enterprise Council (BREC).

The studies should explore different mechanisms for implementing a 3-year cap on support from RPGs, as well as expansion of funding mechanisms to provide researchers who have demonstrated the capacity and inclination for an academic research career, with additional but limited time to complete their research projects and secure an academic appointment. The committee is aware that the current number of postdoctoral awards is grossly insufficient to support postdoctoral researchers who would, under the suggested 3-year cap, be required to transition from RPGs. An additional and serious complication relates to the current restrictions on the capacity of foreign postdoctoral researchers to be supported on F-type training fellowships, T-type institutional training grants, or K-type mentored career awards, with the exception of the K99/R00 Pathway to Independence award. Currently, 53 percent of the postdoctoral researchers at U.S. academic institutions[16] are not eli-

---

[16] See https://ncsesdata.nsf.gov/gradpostdoc/2015/html/GSS2015_DST_47.html (accessed February 9, 2019).

gible for support on federal fellowships and training grants. If the eligibility criteria are not changed, then the imposition of a 3-year cap on support from RPGs would deprive the enterprise of access to a large and outstanding cadre of talent and would have a devastating impact on the quality of the current workforce.

Therefore, prior to implementation of a 3-year cap, along with the pilot studies, there should be action on Recommendation 4.2, that is, to increase the numbers of individual F- and K-type awards that are not restricted to U.S. citizens and permanent residents. In addition, there should be a transitional period between the last fellowship decision received by a postdoctoral researcher and termination of their support on an RPG.

The committee remands to NIH the responsibility of developing any additional steps that are necessary to effectively shift postdoctoral researchers from funding on RPGs to fellowships at the end of 3 years. These steps could include expansion in the number or eligibility of certain other existing awards and creation of a new award tailored to the needs of this population. The model of a temporally phased approach to postdoctoral training presents an opportunity to experiment with entirely new modes of funding, and the committee encourages NIH to make ample use of this opportunity.[17]

More generally, in designing the proposed pilot study, NIH should consider the many complexities that may arise with implementation of a new cap of this type. These may include, but are not limited to

- the implications for PIs, including, in particular, the potential for a negative impact on newly established and resource-limited laboratories and ESIs;
- the consequences of imposing rigid timing constraints for independent research career progression, especially for underrepresented groups, including women, ethnic minorities, and persons with disabilities;
- the potential to favor incremental or conservative research over more innovative proposals if postdoctoral researchers must compete successfully for fellowships in their second year;
- the potential for an adverse effect on internationally trained Ph.D.'s; and
- the consequences of differential overhead rates on research grants versus fellowship (F-type) and career development (K-type) awards.

If due care is not taken in addressing these issues, widespread and consistent imposition of the cap could very well harm the populations that this recommendation is intended to benefit—especially ESIs and individuals already underrepresented in the biomedical research fields. At any rate, the need for careful

---

[17] The committee debated the development of a new 3-year award (with a 2-year extension) that would be portable for use anywhere in the biomedical research enterprise—academia, government (intramural or other government research institution), big pharma/biotech, or small business—providing that the training has a strong research component.

consideration of these issues is precisely why the recommended pilot studies are important instruments for stimulating evidence-based changes in the country's complex biomedical research enterprise.

Finally, Recommendation 4.4 endorses recommendations from earlier reports that postdoctoral training on any funding mechanism be limited to 5 years (Appendix B). After 5 years, any postdoctoral researcher continuing in the same laboratory should be shifted to employment as a staff scientist with an increase in salary and benefits appropriate for a permanent staff member. However, postdoctoral researchers should be allowed to request a short extension beyond the 5 years to account for unplanned circumstances or parental responsibilities.

Taken together, these recommendations seek to engage an enduring concern, one expressed in numerous earlier reports, that most postdoctoral researchers are supported for extended periods of time on RPGs that do not adequately promote their mentorship, training, or transition to independence. RPGs enable the PI to use postdoctoral researchers as technicians who are expected to execute predefined aims. Under these conditions, many postdoctoral researchers face barriers to cultivating independence. It was not always this way; the percentage of postdoctoral researchers supported on these mechanisms has skyrocketed in recent years. These recommendations seek to ease the postdoctoral research population away from this funding mechanism.

While acknowledging all of these complexities and their diverse opinions about the potential implications of these recommendations, the committee members were unanimous in the belief that the postdoctoral experience should be considered a period of mentored transition to independence and that an enforceable, innovative, and tested mechanism is necessary to promote the career progression to independent careers. Previous recommendations have fallen short of stimulating the action needed to transform this crucial career stage. The system is now primed for innovative, rather than incremental, systemic change—if done deliberately and with care.

CREATE OPPORTUNITIES FOR ENTREPRENEURIAL ACTIVITY

Recommendation 4.5
Congress and the National Institutes of Health (NIH) should create and expand existing entrepreneurial and private-sector opportunities to attract and support the next generation of biomedical and behavioral researchers.

- **Congress should revise the Small Business Innovation Research (SBIR)/Small Business Technology Transfer (STTR) program to enable NIH to create a novel ecosystem that fosters entrepreneurship for next generation biomedical scientists, facilitates women- and minority-owned entrepreneurship, and supports fulfillment of NIH's mission across the private sector.**

- Congress should extend/establish an employment tax credit to research and development (R&D) firms for hiring recently minted Ph.D.'s, M.D.'s, and M.D.-Ph.D.'s. and make the credit higher for small- to medium-sized R&D firms and firms that recruit into R&D activity for the first time.

One avenue for creating additional opportunities for Ph.D.'s, M.D.'s, and M.D.-Ph.D.'s to pursue independent research careers outside of academia would be an individual grant mechanism geared toward promoting entrepreneurship in the small business environment. Small business has long been recognized as "critical to the nation's economic strength, to building America's future, and to helping the United States compete in today's global marketplace."[18] In 1982, Congress created the Small Business Innovation Research (SBIR) program to encourage small businesses to develop new processes and products and to provide quality research in support of the U.S. government's missions. In 1992 it created the Small Business Technology Transfer (STTR) program to expand partnership opportunities for small business and nonprofit research institutions by requiring small business recipients to collaborate with academic research institutions.[19] The SBIR/STTR program is overseen by an interagency committee co-chaired by the White House Office of Science and Technology and Policy and the Small Business Administration, and it is implemented through 11 federal agencies, including the Department of Health and Human Services (HHS). In 2015, HHS awarded $813.8 million in SBIR/STTR funds, with the majority provided by NIH.[20]

In light of the 2016 21st Century Cures Act[21] and 2017 American Innovation and Competitiveness Act,[22] which includes a focus on the next generation of researchers and the promotion of scientific entrepreneurship, the committee examined whether the central structure of the SBIR/STTR program as implemented by HHS should be modified to align with the goals of those laws. The development of programs and support mechanisms that encourage early-career researchers to engage with the small business enterprise can provide critical preparation for biomedical research trainees, including postdoctoral researchers, to become biomedical innovators and advance economic growth. To achieve this endpoint, the NIH SBIR/STTR program should be modified to enable grants/contracts to small businesses that aim to reduce the cost of research. Several models for this approach exist across other federal agencies that participate in the SBIR program.

Mechanisms already exist within the SBIR/STTR program portfolio to engage early-career researchers. One such example is the Small Business Postdoctoral Research Diversity Fellowship Program supported by the National

---

[18] See https://www.sba.gov/about-sba/what-we-do/mission (accessed December 6, 2017).
[19] See https://www.sbir.gov/tutorials/program-basics/tutorial-5 (accessed February 9, 2018).
[20] See https://www.sbir.gov/awards/annual-reports?view_by=Agency (accessed December 6, 2017).
[21] 21st Century Cures Act, P.L. 114-225, 130 Stat. 1033-1344 (2016).
[22] American Innovation and Competitiveness Act, P.L. 114-329, 130 Stat. 2969-3038 (2017).

Science Foundation (NSF),[23] which promotes the engagement of postdoctoral researchers from underrepresented groups in NSF-supported SBIR companies. Congress and NIH should build on that precedent by adapting other mechanisms not currently linked to the SBIR/STIR program to promote entrepreneurship in the next generation of researchers. For example, a mechanism similar to the NIH Pathways to Independence Award (K99/R00) could be developed within the SBIR program to provide mentoring for early-career scientists and aids their transition to independence within the small business ecosystem, rather than academia. In the same way, a model similar to the Research Supplements to Promote Diversity in Health-Related Research program, which provides earmarked funding for established scientists to mentor diverse trainees interested in pursuing careers in health-related research, could be developed within the SBIR/STTR program to promote diversity in the small business-driven ecosystem.

A separate avenue for cultivating independent research opportunities for talented biomedical trainees and creating more opportunities for them in the private sector would require Congress to extend or establish an employment tax credit for R&D firms that hire new Ph.D.'s, M.D.'s, and M.D.-Ph.D.'s. By lowering the cost of hiring researchers, a tax credit should stimulate employment in R&D. The tax credit recommendation builds on Action D-2 from the National Research Council report *Rising Above the Gathering Storm* (National Academy of Sciences et al., 2007, p. 11) to "enact a stronger research and development tax credit to encourage private investment in innovation."

The logic for the tax credit rests on two facts. First, tax credits are more effective when the supply of labor is forthcoming without an accompanying increase in wages (Bartik and Bishop, 2009). Second, tax credits in the form of wage subsidies for Ph.D.'s have been found to have a positive effect on the number of Ph.D. researchers hired by Belgian firms (Dumont, 2015). They have also been shown to be effective in stimulating R&D hiring by firms that have previously not engaged in research (Neicu et al., 2016). Moreover, the tax credit provides opportunities to target certain types of firms. By way of example, and consistent with the recommendation designed to stimulate entrepreneurial activity on the part of recently trained biomedical researchers, the credit could be higher for small- to medium-sized R&D firms or for young innovative companies. Such a policy would be similar to one in Belgium that provides a tax exemption on wage subsidies associated with recruiting and hiring scientists for young innovative companies and research organizations (Dumont, 2015).

REFERENCES

Bankston, A., and G. S. McDowell. 2017. Monitoring the compliance of the academic enterprise with the Fair Labor Standards Act. *F1000Research* 5:2690. https://f1000research.com/articles/5-2690/v2 (accessed February 8, 2018)

---

[23] See https://nsfsbir.asee.org/ (accessed December 6, 2017).

Bartik, T. J., and J. H. Bishop. 2009. *The job creation tax credit: Dismal projections for employment call for a quick, efficient, and effective response*. Washington, DC: Economic Policy Institute.

Dumont, M. 2015. *Evaluation of federal tax incentives for private R&D in Belgium: An update*. Brussels: Federal Planning Bureau.

Gibbs, K. D., J. McGready, and K. Griffin. 2015. Career development among American biomedical postdocs. *CBE Life Sciences Education* 14(4):ar44.

Institute of Medicine, National Academy of Sciences, and National Academy of Engineering. 2000. *Enhancing the postdoctoral experience for scientists and engineers: A guide for postdoctoral scholars, advisers, institutions, funding organizations, and disciplinary societies*. Washington, DC: The National Academies Press.

Kahn, S., and D. K. Ginther. 2017. The impact of postdoctoral training on early careers in biomedicine. *Nature Biotechnology* 35(1):90-94.

National Academy of Sciences, National Academy of Engineering, and Institute of Medicine. 2007. *Rising above the gathering storm: Energizing and employing America for a brighter economic future*. Washington, DC: The National Academies Press.

National Academy of Sciences, National Academy of Engineering, and Institute of Medicine. 2014. *The postdoctoral experience revisited*. Washington, DC: The National Academies Press.

National Institutes of Health. 2012. *Biomedical research workforce working group report*. Bethesda, MD: National Institutes of Health.

National Research Council. 2005. *Bridges to independence: Fostering the independence of new investigators in biomedical research*. Washington, DC: The National Academies Press.

Neicu, D., P. Teirlinck, and S. Kelchtermans. 2016. Dipping in the policy mix: Do R&D subsidies foster behavioral additionality effects of R&D tax credits? *Economics of Innovation and New Technology* 25(3):218-239.

Sauermann, H., and M. Roach. 2012. Science PhD career preferences: Levels, changes, and advisor encouragement. *PloS One* 7(5):e36307.

Working Group on Diversity in the Biomedical Research Workforce. 2012. *Draft report of the Advisory Committee to the Director: Working Group on Diversity in the Biomedical Research Workforce*. Bethesda, MD: National Institutes of Health.

5

Building a Better Ecosystem for Independence

Chapter 2 chronicled the challenges that early-career investigators face as they transition to and sustain research independence. In this chapter, the committee identifies a series of reforms to the existing biomedical[1] ecosystem designed to create stronger and more easily navigable pathways to independent research opportunities for investigators regardless of gender, race, ethnicity, sexual orientation, socioeconomic background, visa status, or degree. If adopted, these reforms would provide stable and supportive platforms for success at each stage in a researcher's career, while ensuring that the most promising candidates proceed to the next stage of training and mentorship and that robust exit opportunities exist for those who choose not to progress to an academic appointment. An ideal ecosystem would strike a balance between low-risk and high-risk lines of research, between basic and applied research, and between opportunities to work independently or as part of a team of independent investigators. It would also provide appropriate mentoring and financial support in a manner that does not place an arbitrary and undue burden on young scientists from any background, but instead creates equitable opportunities for all qualified investigators to succeed.

As highlighted in commissioned papers by international contributors,[2] the U.S. biomedical research ecosystem is not unique in the challenges facing younger investigators or in its desire to attract and retain the best and the brightest in rewarding research careers. Canada, for example, has been working to rejuvenate its biomedical research workforce in the face of declining federal research funds and increasing pressures on entry-level academic positions resulting from

---

[1] In this report, "biomedical" refers to the full range of biological, biomedical, behavioral, and health sciences supported by the National Institutes of Health.

[2] See http://www.nas.edu/NextGen/Commissioned (accessed February 22, 2018).

an end to mandatory retirement in universities and colleges. The European Union is grappling with its own misalignment between the supply of and demand for trainees, availability of faculty positions, and the need to train young scientists for diverse careers. The countries that provided input to the committee are addressing many issues similar to those experienced in the United States:

- whether to allocate additional funds set aside for early-career investigators;
- whether to increase the size and duration of funding for these investigators;
- how to avoid unintended consequences for mid-career investigators seeking follow-on funding; and
- how to monitor success of these populations in systems under stress.

The committee strongly endorsed the urgent need to solve the persistent and severe structural issues described in Chapter 2 that impact early-career investigators. These issues command deliberate attention from and action by all stakeholders, including the federal government, academic and research institutions, and industries in the biomedical space. The committee's recommendations are predicated on the strong belief that collaboration from all stakeholders will be required to strengthen the system in the manner envisaged by this committee.

Recommendation 5.1
The National Institutes of Health (NIH) should invest in strengthening the research funding landscape for the next generation of investigators.

- **To promote innovative research with high potential for groundbreaking discoveries, NIH should expand the number of NIH Director's New Innovator Awards (DP2) and similar programs funded by individual NIH Institutes and Centers.**
- **NIH should ensure that the duration of all R01 research grants supporting early-stage investigators (ESIs) is no less than 5 years to enable the establishment of resilient independent research programs. NIH Institutes and Centers should monitor the effect of this change on the availability of funds for other research project grants and should experiment with further extensions of the duration of R01 awards for ESIs.**
- **To avoid dis-incentivizing research collaboration, those ESIs who participate in multi-principal investigator (PI) submissions prior to receiving their own R01 grants should retain their ESI status unless serving as a co-PI on a funded multi-PI award provides them with R01-equivalent funds for their own research.**
- **NIH should expand the Pathways to Independence (K99/R00) award, with a priority on fostering independence through career development, including the development of an innovative and independent**

research project originally conceived of and executed by the applicant, rather than additional or new training.

The committee strongly supports NIH's recent announcement of the Next Generation Researchers Initiative (NGRI) and encourages Congress to allocate new funds to support this initiative. NIH should evaluate on a regular basis its new programs with the goal of expanding those that prove effective at addressing the challenges that ESIs and early established investigators (EEIs) face as they attempt to become independent investigators. The committee also commends NIH's support of ESIs who pursue R01 awards through previous ESI-specific policies, including preferential paylines and segregated review. These efforts have had a positive impact on the success rates for the intended applicant pools (see Figure 2-4).

In the past, most R01-equivalent grants were funded for 5 years, but the duration and number of R01 awards have decreased as the number of applicants has increased out of proportion to the NIH budget. Initial NIH funding for ESIs should be long enough in duration and large enough in amount to support establishment of new, independent research programs. We recommend 5 years and at least $250,000 per year of direct cost. Furthermore, NIH should consider exempting the first R01 for ESIs from administrative cuts after the grant is awarded so that those investigators are not penalized as they establish their programs.

In 2007, NIH unveiled the DP2 to support highly innovative research from exceptionally creative ESIs. DP2 applicants can request up to $1.5 million in direct costs over the 5-year grant period. Although the DP2 award appears to be an excellent mechanism to support ESIs who plan innovative projects, NIH expects to make only 33 awards in 2018, depending on the availability of funds in the NIH Common Fund.[3] Given that the DP2 award has successfully motivated early-career investigators to propose and conduct innovative, high-risk, and impactful biomedical and bio-behavioral research, NIH should encourage Institutes and Centers to implement similar mechanisms, such as the National Institute of Mental Health (NIMH)'s Biobehavioral Research Awards for Innovative New Investigators (R01) award. Many organizations that responded to the Dear Colleague Letter (Appendix C) strongly urged expansion of the DP2 program. The committee requests that NIH expand the number of DP2 awards and mount a pilot project to determine whether there are tangible advantages to increasing the duration of the DP2 and similar awards, such as the National Institute of Neurological Disorders and Stroke's Research Program (R35) award with an 8-year duration, the National Cancer Institute (NCI)'s Outstanding Investigator Award (R35) with a 7-year duration, and the National Institutes of General Medical Science's MERIT (R37) award with a potential 8- to 10- year duration. The benefits could include, but are not limited to, higher success rates for securing subsequent NIH

---

[3] See http://grants.nih.gov/grants/guide/rfa-files/RFA-RM-17-006.html (accessed March 21, 2018).

awards, increased publication and citation rates, or increased willingness to undertake higher risk research.

In 2006, NIH established the NIH K99/R00 award to "help outstanding postdoctoral researchers with a research and/or clinical doctorate degree complete needed, mentored career development and transition in a timely manner to independent, tenure-track or equivalent faculty positions."[4] Recipients of the K99/R00 award have been found to have a higher success rate for subsequent R01-equivalent awards compared to new ESIs and are more persistent in obtaining subsequent grant support (Carlson et al., 2016). In addition, a 2014 analysis by Grantome found that close to 60 percent of 2007 K99 awardees became the PI on a research project grant (RPG), compared to less than 20 percent for postdocs supported on F32 awards (Grantome, 2014). The committee commends NIH for developing a program that artfully connects training and independence, and recommends that NIH consider expanding this program with some modifications, such as extending the length of the R00 portion of the grant beyond 3 years, ceasing funding of applicable indirect costs from the R00 portion of the grant,[5] and decreasing the emphasis on the new/additional training component of the K99 proposal.

Recommendation 5.2
The National Institutes of Health (NIH) should continue to improve the peer review process to optimize the evaluation of applications submitted by early-stage and early experienced investigators in the Next Generation Researchers Initiative. This action would especially benefit investigators from underrepresented groups. NIH should revise the biosketch requirement to focus peer review on recent contributions and accomplishments and should continue to test effective practices to reduce the effects of implicit bias on the review process and to increase the diversity of reviewers.

Traditionally, a young investigator's receipt of an initial R01 or equivalent award has been viewed as a marker of early independence and success. However, data suggest that ESIs experience difficulties in the peer review process that may disadvantage them compared to established investigators (Azoulay et al., 2013). In 2008, NIH issued a report that addressed many issues surrounding peer review (National Institutes of Health, 2008). In that report, NIH assessed that some policies, such as the single resubmission policy, disproportionately disadvantage newer investigators because they tend to have smaller research programs and facilities. The committee supports the need for additional action to reduce the barriers that ESIs face in the grant review process. Although adjustment of paylines has assisted, other measures can improve the review and success of ESI applications.

---

[4] See https://grants.nih.gov/grants/guide/pa-files/PA-16-077.html (accessed March 20, 2018).

[5] The current R00 award is up to $249,000 total costs per year, including salary, research support, and indirect costs.

To improve the review process for ESIs, NIH identifies ESI applications when they are assigned to a study section so that appropriate consideration of career stage can be applied during review. To facilitate this effort, ESI applications are clustered, or reviewed together, to enable evaluation as a group, and NIH instructs peer reviewers to focus more on the proposed approach than on the track record and to expect less preliminary data than might be provided by an established investigator.

NIH requires a standardized biosketch to accompany every grant application. The biosketch highlights an individual's qualifications for the proposed research project. In the current application format, applicants describe their major contributions and list four to five publications that reflect each contribution. Since the current biosketch format focuses on the totality of the researcher's career, and places less emphasis on recent productivity, it could advantage more established over younger investigators in the review process.

Revising the biosketch requirement to emphasize recent productivity could help to level the playing field for ESIs. Canada adopted a similar approach, whereby applicants for Natural Sciences and Engineering Research Council (NSERC) grants are assessed on the quality and impact of their contributions to research over the past 6 years instead of the duration of their careers.[6]

All investigators, but particularly ESIs, would benefit from increased diversity on the review panels. The committee also recommends that NIH expand the number of junior investigators who serve as ad hoc members on review committees and afford them an opportunity to learn more about the peer review process. In addition, NIH should continue to develop training strategies to address implicit biases in peer review. Data reveal that grants submitted by members of underrepresented minority groups (Ginther et al., 2011) receive lower priority scores than those submitted by their white counterparts. The committee applauds NIH for its current efforts and notes that current studies are under way to identify effective remediation strategies.[7] The committee requests quick dissemination of these studies' findings and full funding of any additional research needed to promote equity during the peer review process.

Recommendation 5.3
Research institutions and the National Institutes of Health should develop mechanisms to increase the number of individuals in staff scientist positions to provide more stable, non-faculty research opportunities for the next generation of researchers. Research institutions should experiment with providing career tracks with clearly defined review and promotion processes, as well as opportunities for professional development. Individuals in a staff

---

[6] See http://www.nserc-crsng.gc.ca/NSERC-CRSNG/Policies-Politiques/assesscontrib-evalcontrib_eng.asp (accessed December 10, 2017).

[7] See https://acd.od.nih.gov/documents/presentations/06082017Valantine.pdf (accessed December 10, 2017).

scientist track should receive a salary and benefits commensurate with their experience and responsibilities.

Relatively few established paths exist for researchers who pursue research at academic institutions as non-faculty researchers, often referred to as staff scientists. These positions often do not include clear opportunities for career advancement, and they rarely allow access to the professional resources available to faculty and trainees. In many cases, staff scientists work in the laboratories of individual PIs and are not encouraged to secure independent research support. In addition, few funding mechanisms are dedicated to supporting professional, non-faculty researchers in academia, and staff scientists who receive an NIH grant find it difficult to sustain their careers because of federal prohibitions against spending time writing grants when they are supported by a federal grant (Carpenter, 2012).

The lack of clarity around established career paths at many universities other than academic faculty positions is a flaw in today's academic biomedical enterprise. This flaw contributes to many of the issues discussed in this report, including the backlog of postdoctoral researchers and confusion and frustration on the part of trainees and PIs. Promotion of a staff scientist track as an attractive and viable research career choice in academia—one with stability and professional recognition and status as well as opportunities for progressive advancement—would provide a career path for individuals who are interested in academic research but are not interested in an academic faculty position. This action would help to bring the biomedical system into greater equilibrium, though it is possible that the increased use of staff scientists could impact the downstream availability of faculty positions, a possibility that will require careful monitoring to avoid.

At many institutions, it is staff scientists who manage the sophisticated research technologies located in core and other shared facilities. These services and technologies are essential to the success of biomedical investigators' endeavors and therefore the overall biomedical research enterprise. Therefore, programs to support a unique class of independent or semi-independent staff scientists are needed. Many will be leaders of scientific core facilities or shared resources, and while they will enjoy a degree of independence, they will nearly always focus on providing collaborative support and making critical research technologies accessible. This recommendation is intended to further the development of a cadre of staff scientists, provide research-based opportunities for academic scientists beyond a faculty research appointment, and support advancement of the nation's biomedical research.

Recognition of the role for staff scientists in the research enterprise is growing. Academic institutions such as the University of Wisconsin-Madison, the Howard Hughes Medical Institute's Janelia Research Campus, the Salk Institute of Biological Sciences, NIH Clinical Center, NIH intramural laboratories, and the Allen Institute for Brain Science have developed formal programs for staff scientists. The Broad Institute is notable for its Institute Scientist initiative and for employing more than 400 staff scientists (Hyman, 2017). In recognition of the key role that staff scientists can play in advancing complex scientific projects, the NCI launched in 2015 a new Research Specialist Award (R50) pilot program for exceptional scientists who want to pursue research within the context of an existing cancer research program, but not serve as independent investigators. The R50 is intended to provide desirable salaries and sufficient autonomy so that individuals are not solely dependent on grants held by PIs for career continuity.

However, meaningful evaluation of the potential impact of staff scientist or equivalent positions will depend on the design of new programs that extend beyond NCI and can fund more than a few dozen positions. This area is well suited for funding experimental pilot projects, and NIH and universities alike should explore development of programs that provide support for original research projects conducted by staff scientists. These programs should be open to qualified scientists regardless of visa status. In addition, institutional leadership will need to nurture an environment that supports staff scientists and attracts high-caliber investigators who want to work in non-faculty academic positions. The nature of pilot projects differs from that of RPGs; therefore, the metrics for their evaluation should be considered carefully. Evaluation criteria should aim to capture the holistic contributions of the scientist and could include contributions to published work noted in authorship, contributorship (Rennie et al., 1997; Sauermann and Haeussler, 2017) or acknowledgement, contributions to data that result in successful grant funding, and the breadth and numbers of different independent researchers that are assisted. In addition, NIH or the National Science Foundation (NSF) should track the career paths of staff scientists in the same ways that this report recommends they track the career paths of postdoctoral researchers (see Recommendation 3.3).

Many of the responses to the Dear Colleague Letter (Appendix C) highlighted the need to better support staff and professional scientists given their contributions to the biomedical research enterprise. Based on the findings of its working group to study the issues confronting staff scientists, the American Society for Biochemistry and Molecular Biology (ASBMB) is planning a study to collect data on the cost, efficiency, and productivity of staff scientists as a means to develop guidance for the research community on how best to incorporate staff scientists into its operations. The ASBMB working group proposed that institutions create individual development plans for staff scientists to ensure they receive some degree of professional development and career advice. In a 2015 report, *Sustaining Discovery* (FASEB, 2015, p. 5), the Federation of American Societies for Experimental Biology (FASEB) called for the research community to employ more staff scientists and to consider more extensive use of career technicians, as have others (Pickett et al., 2015).

Recommendation 5.4
The National Institutes of Health (NIH), research institutions, and principal investigators should share responsibility for increasing diversity and promoting inclusion of early-career researchers.

- To promote diversity and inclusion at the junior faculty level, NIH should require an institutional diversity and inclusion plan as a component of the institutional resources reported on research grants supporting trainees.
- To promote diversity and inclusion of research trainees, principal investigators should provide a diversity and inclusion plan in their grant proposals and should provide updates in progress reports, if funded.

The ability of science to promote worldwide health and prosperity requires a culture that supports and sustains a diverse and innovative biomedical workforce, but recent studies suggest that women—particularly women of color—and individuals from underrepresented populations (Hispanic or Latino, African American, American Indian and Alaska Native) experience higher rates of attrition in the transition from Ph.D. to academic faculty positions (Gibbs et al., 2014, 2016). Research into why improvements in gender, race, and ethnicity representation at the doctoral level are not reflected at the postdoctoral researcher and faculty career stages is ongoing, as is research on how best to restructure training, mentoring, and faculty hiring practices to reverse this trend.

One obvious priority is to address concerns about the effect of current hiring, tenure, and promotion policies on diversity and inclusion. These concerns arise from evidence-based observations about the enduring challenge of increasing faculty diversity. The first observation from recent studies is that the improved diversity in the ranks of trainees has not carried forward to the ranks of tenured professors (Finkelstein et al., 2016; Gibbs et al., 2016; Li and Koedel, 2017). At most academic medical centers, for example, promotion rates for African American and Hispanic faculty were lower than those for their non-Hispanic white peers (Nunez-Smith et al., 2012). In one set of studies in European countries, where faculty tenure and promotion decisions are made by randomly assigned committees, the promotion chances of female candidates for faculty promotion were diminished if they were assigned to an all-male review committee rather than a mixed-gender review committee (De Paola and Scoppa, 2015; Zinovyeva and Bagues, 2010).

Establishing institution-wide and laboratory-specific diversity and inclusion plans would go a long way in encouraging research institutions and their PIs to participate actively in addressing underrepresentation in the scientific research workforce. The committee applauds the National Institute of General Medical Sciences' recently announced plans to require institutions to report evidence-based diversity and inclusion approaches in all T32 proposals and to include these plans as part of scored review criteria. Such initiatives would encourage institutions to develop their own official diversity and inclusion plans and strategies that investigators can leverage when recruiting and training students and postdoctoral researchers.

Recommendation 5.5
The National Institutes of Health should allocate funds from its Next Generation Researchers Initiative to expand the number of Research Supplements to Promote Diversity in Health-Related Research (PA-16-288). These should be awarded to underrepresented minority (URM) early-stage investigators and URM investigators who have not been awarded a research project grant and seek to collaborate with funded investigators on new but related research projects. Proposals must clearly detail how the collaboration will result in a grant proposal by the URM investigator. To best support this career stage, awards should be enhanced with funds for supplies, equipment, professional development, and mentoring. The eligibility criteria for these diversity supplements should reflect only the URM populations specified by the National Science Foundation for the biomedical research enterprise.

In response to the 21st Century Cures Act of 2016,[8] NIH launched the Next Generation Research Initiative (NGRI). This policy established ESIs and EEIs as two classes of scientists that would be prioritized for funding. In replacing the 2007 NIH New Investigator policy, the NGRI increases the possibility of unintended consequences from enhancing workforce diversity specifically within the biomedical research enterprise as called for by the 21st Century Cures Act. The NIH Research Supplements to Promote Diversity in Health-Related Research program can be utilized as part of the NGRI to counterbalance these potential unintended consequences.

Currently, only 10 percent of all diversity supplements are used to support faculty-level investigators (Valantine et al., 2016). As part of an NIH-wide program, PIs on RPGs may request supplemental funds to support and recruit eligible investigators from underrepresented racial and ethnic groups and with disabilities. Individuals who meet the criteria for "Investigators Developing Independent Research Careers" as specified in the solicitation can receive up to 2 years of funding and $10,000 for travel and supplies. As part of the NGRI, this support should be increased to provide up to 3 years of salary support ($75,000/ year maximum) and $50,000/year for supplies and travel.

The National Institute of Neurological Disorders and Stroke (NINDS), responding to its assessment of its diversity supplement program, instituted

---

[8] 21st Century Cures Act, P.L. 114-225 § 2021, 130 Stat. 1051, 1052 (2016). Available at https://www.congress.gov/114/bills/hr34/BILLS-114hr34enr.pdf (accessed January 19, 2018).

rigorous review criteria and now requires the student or fellow supported by a diversity supplement to write an individual proposal within 2 years of receipt of support from this program. This approach should be extended to Next Generation Researchers Initiative-Diversity Supplements (NGRI-DS).

The eligibility criteria for administrative supplements has been the subject of debate. The committee recommends limiting the eligibility for underrepresented racial and ethnic groups to those groups underrepresented in science, technology, engineering, and mathematics (STEM) fields as defined by NSF. The committee also recommends that eligibility for the NGRI-DS should not extend to individuals from economically or educationally disadvantaged backgrounds unless evidence demonstrates that this group is at a competitive disadvantage during the ESI and EEI stages.

Recommendation 5.6
The National Institutes of Health (NIH) should make the Loan Repayment Programs available to all individuals pursuing biomedical physician-scientist researcher careers, regardless of their research area or clinical specialty. NIH should increase the monetary value of loan repayment to reflect the debt burden of current medical trainees. NIH should also continue implementation of the recommendations laid out in the 2014 NIH *Physician-Scientist Workforce Working Group Report*. NIH should test new strategies and expand effective approaches to increase the pool of early-stage physician-scientists.

Physician-scientists function as a critical segment of the biomedical research workforce because they bridge the clinical and research enterprises and thus help to accelerate the translation of basic discoveries into medical advances. In addition to the challenges that all ESIs face, physician-scientists face some unique challenges early in their research careers. For example, the training required to obtain competency in clinical and scientific research is extensive, and, not surprisingly, achieving proficiency in both can require a long overall training period. In addition, physician-scientists face increasing clinical demands, thereby decreasing their time for investigative work. In the face of these challenges, additional incentives are needed to support clinicians interested in either pursuing or sustaining their research programs (NIH Physician Scientist Workforce Working Group, 2014).

Initiatives such NIH's Loan Repayment Programs (LRP) for physician-scientists are helpful in encouraging research activity by physician-scientists, but the program has not kept pace with the increasing cost of medical school and is only available in some biomedical fields. As of 2017, NIH's LRP will pay 25 percent of the eligible education debt up to a maximum of $35,000 of loan repayment per year, with an option for a 1- or 2-year renewal. However, the median medical school debt in 2016 was $190,000, a nearly $20,000 increase since 2011,[9] and the loan repayment amount is considered taxable income. Division of Loan Repayment at NIH pays federal taxes for the LRP recipient on a quarterly basis at 39 percent of the loan repayment. However the LRP recipient may be subject to other taxes such as state taxes. In fiscal year 2017, this program made 1,283 awards totaling $68,185,910. With 74 percent of medical school graduates from 2016 with education debt,[10] physicians are less likely to pursue biomedical research and become physician-scientists than they were in the past (Garrison and Deschamps, 2014).

In 2016, the 21st Century Cures Act authorized increases in the amount of loan forgiveness to a maximum of $50,000 per year and granted the NIH Director authority to expand the number of repayments to reflect workforce and research needs. However, NIH has not yet expanded LRP access for physician-scientists beyond the current programs for which they are eligible: clinical research, pediatric research, health disparities research, contraception and infertility research, and clinical research for individuals from disadvantaged backgrounds. Therefore, the committee recommends that NIH make the LRP available to all individuals pursuing biomedical physician-scientist researcher careers, regardless of their research area or clinical specialty, and that NIH increase the dollar amount of loans forgiven to reflect the debt burden of current medical trainees to incentivize talented physicians to pursue independent biomedical research careers.

Ensuring that physician-scientists have dedicated time for research, as well as adequate mentoring, is perhaps the most effective intervention to retaining young academic medical faculty in the NIH workforce. Time devoted to clinical care and financial pressures are strong predictors of attrition (Dzirasa et al., 2015; Lingard et al., 2017; Milewicz et al., 2015; Turner, 2012). Career mentoring and peer support have been identified as effective measures for supporting young physician-scientists, particularly among women and underrepresented minorities (Byington et al., 2016; Chen et al., 2016; Dzirasa et al., 2015; Gotian et al., 2017).

Prompted by the 2014 *NIH Physician-Scientist Workforce Report*, NIH has begun to explore several approaches to support physician-scientists, such as decreasing the length of training, reducing educational debt, and encouraging earlier mentored-research experiences. One example of such a program is the new National Heart, Lung, and Blood Institute Stimulating Access to Research in Residency R38 research program.[11] This program funds qualifying institutions to provide outstanding mentored research opportunities to resident-investigators and to foster their ability to transition to individual career development research awards. The program enables institutions to provide support for up to 2 years of

---

[9] See https://news.aamc.org/medical-education/article/taking-sting-out-medical-school-debt/ (accessed December 15, 2017).

[10] See https://www.lrp.nih.gov/ (accessed December 15, 2017).

[11] See https://grants.nih.gov/grants/guide/rfa-files/RFA-HL-18-023.html (accessed December 15, 2017).

research conducted by resident-investigators in structured programs for clinician-investigators with defined program milestones.

In 2017, NINDS established the Neurosurgeon Research Career Development (K12) Award,[12] with the goal of expanding the cadre of neurosurgeon investigators trained to conduct research into neurological disorders. The K12 award provides 5 years of funding to research organizations to support a national research career development program. Although this K12 award is housed at the program director (PD)'s or PI's institution, it is not intended to support scholars solely at that institution. The PD/PI can solicit applications from eligible candidates at institutions from across the country, and selected scholars will proceed with their career development and research plan at their home institution, with a local mentor. The committee encourages NIH to continue piloting programs and institutions to not only participate actively in these programs but also develop and test their own innovative programs. When successful, NIH should encourage every Institute and Center to adopt such programs.

Some academic institutions have established innovative programs to help researchers dedicate more time to research and increase their productivity. Harvard Medical School's Office for Diversity Inclusion and Community Partnership Faculty Fellowship,[13] for example, provides junior faculty with 2 years of fellowship support in the amount of $50,000 per year to release time from clinical work to conduct an individual, mentored research project. NIH could incentivize these types of efforts by providing matching flexible funds to institutions that are exploring ways to retain physician-scientists. The funds could be used to protect research time or to provide mentoring services.

REFERENCES

Azoulay, P., J. Graff Zivin, and G. Manso. 2013. National Institutes of Health peer review: Challenges and avenues for reform. *Innovation Policy and the Economy* 13(1):1-22.

Byington, C. L., H. Keenan, J. D. Phillips, R. Childs, E. Wachs, M. A. Berzins, K. Clark, M. K. Torres, J. Abramson, V. Lee, and E. B. Clark. 2016. A matrix mentoring model that effectively supports clinical and translational scientists and increases inclusion in biomedical research: Lessons from the University of Utah. *Academic Medicine* 91(4):497-502.

Carlson, D. E., W. C. Wang, and J. D. Scott. 2016. Initial outcomes for the NHLBI K99/R00 pathway to independence program in relation to long-standing career development programs: Implications for trainees, mentors, and institutions. *Circulation Research* 119(8):904-908.

Carpenter, S. 2012. A hidden academic workforce. In *Share*. Science Magazine website: American Association for the Advancement of Science.

Chen, M. M., C. I. Sandborg, L. Hudgins, R. Sanford, and L. K. Bachrach. 2016. A multifaceted mentoring program for junior faculty in academic pediatrics. *Teaching and Learning in Medicine* 28(3):320-328.

De Paola, M., and V. Scoppa. 2015. Gender discrimination and evaluators' gender: Evidence from Italian academia. *Economica* 82(325):162-188.

---

[12] See https://grants.nih.gov/grants/guide/rfa-files/RFA-NS-17-010.html (accessed February 9, 2018).

[13] See https://mfdp.med.harvard.edu/DICP_Faculty_Fellowship (accessed February 9, 2018).

Dzirasa, K., R. R. Krishnan, and R. S. Williams. 2015. Incubating the research independence of a medical scientist training program graduate: A case study. *Academic Medicine* 90(2):176-179.

FASEB (Federation of American Societies for Experimental Biology). 2015. *Sustaining discovery in biological and medical sciences: A framework for discussion.* Bethesda, MD: Federation of American Societies for Experimental Biology.

Finkelstein, M. J., V. M. Conley, and J. H. Schuster. 2016. *Taking the measure of faculty diversity.* New York, NY: TIAA Institute.

Garrison, H. H., and A. M. Deschamps. 2014. NIH research funding and early career physician scientists: Continuing challenges in the 21st century. *FASEB Journal* 28(3):1049-1058.

Gibbs, K. D., Jr., J. McGready, J. C. Bennett, and K. Griffin. 2014. Biomedical science Ph.D. career interest patterns by race/ethnicity and gender. *PloS One* 9(12):e114736.

Gibbs, K. D., J. Basson, I. M. Xierali, and D. A. Broniatowski. 2016. Decoupling of the minority PhD talent pool and assistant professor hiring in medical school basic science departments in the US. *Elife* 5.

Ginther, D. K., W. T. Schaffer, J. Schnell, B. Masimore, F. Liu, L. L. Haak, and R. Kington. 2011. Race, ethnicity, and NIH research awards. *Science* 333(6045):1015-1019.

Gotian, R., J. C. Raymore, S. K. Rhooms, L. Liberman, and O. S. Andersen. 2017. Gateways to the laboratory: How an MD-PhD program increased the number of minority physician-scientists. *Academic Medicine* 92(5):628-634.

Grantome. 2014. In it to win it. In *Grantome*. Cleveland, OH: Grantome.

Hyman, S. 2017. Biology needs more staff scientists. *Nature* 545(7654):283-284.

Li, D., and C. Koedel. 2017. Representation and salary gaps by race-ethnicity and gender at selective public universities. *Educational Researcher* 46(7):343-354.

Lingard, L., P. Zhang, M. Strong, M. Steele, J. Yoo, and J. Lewis. 2017. Strategies for supporting physician-scientists in faculty roles: A narrative review with key informant consultations. *Academic Medicine* 92(10):1421-1428.

Milewicz, D. M., R. G. Lorenz, T. S. Dermody, and L. F. Brass. 2015. Rescuing the physician-scientist workforce: The time for action is now. *Journal of Clinical Investigation* 125(10):3742-3747.

National Institutes of Health. 2008. *National Institutes of Health 2007-2008 peer review self-study.* Bethesda, MD: National Institutes of Health.

NIH Physician Scientist Workforce Working Group. 2014. *Physician Scientist Workforce Working Group report.* Bethesda, MD: National Institutes of Health.

Nunez-Smith, M., M. M. Ciarleglio, T. Sandoval-Schaefer, J. Elumn, L. Castillo-Page, P. Peduzzi, and E. H. Bradley. 2012. Institutional variation in the promotion of racial/ethnic minority faculty at US medical schools. *American Journal of Public Health* 102(5):852-858.

Pickett, C. L., B. W. Corb, C. R. Matthews, W. I. Sundquist, and J. M. Berg. 2015. Toward a sustainable biomedical research enterprise: Finding consensus and implementing recommendations. *Proceedings of the National Academy of Sciences* 112(35):10832-10836.

Rennie, D., V. Yank, and L. Emanuel. 1997. When authorship fails. A proposal to make contributors accountable. *JAMA* 278(7):579-585.

Sauermann, H., and C. Haeussler. 2017. Authorship and contribution disclosures. *Science Advances* 3(11).

Turner, J. R. 2012. Continuing attrition of physician-scientists (caps): A preventable syndrome? *Gastroenterology* 143(3):511-515.e1.

Valantine, H. A., P. K. Lund, and A. E. Gammie. 2016. From the NIH: A systems approach to increasing the diversity of the biomedical research workforce. *CBE Life Sciences Education* 15(3).

Zinovyeva, N., and M. Bagues. 2010. Does gender matter for academic promotion? Evidence from a randomized natural experiment. SSRN, https://ssrn.com/abstract=1618256 (accessed February 19, 2018).

6

Experimentation and Innovation

A system as vast and complex as the biomedical research enterprise requires careful and evidence-based policy solutions. Without a culture of innovation, experimentation, and rigorous assessment, institutions will feel less comfortable adopting policy recommendations, the recommendations that are adopted may be less effective or produce unforeseen consequences, and even the successful ones may not be broadly adopted by institutions over time. And yet, the committee was surprised by the small number of publicly reported, evidence-based studies of the many ideas to address the issues confronting the nation's young investigators, as well as the lack of a site analogous to clinicaltrials.gov to register experiments and pilots of the type mentioned throughout this report. If the nation hopes to design and sustain effective policies to support the next generation of investigators, we need to hardwire into the biomedical research enterprise[1] a greater capacity for experimentation in policy and funding changes, followed by assessment, publication, and adaptation or replication if successful. This is, in essence, how science itself proceeds.

Indeed, many of the responses to the committee's Dear Colleague Letter (see Appendix C) expressed a desire for more experimentation and assessment with public disclosure on approaches to address the challenges identified in this report. For example, the Public Affairs Advisory Committee of the American Society for Biochemistry and Molecular Biology noted that concrete data on the effect of supporting more staff scientists are not readily available and that "understanding the true financial and productivity effects of employing staff scientists would

---

[1] In this report, "biomedical" refers to the full range of biological, biomedical, behavioral, and health sciences supported by the National Institutes of Health.

guide the community on how best to incorporate staff scientists" into their research enterprise. The Association of American Medical Colleges urged that any changes to the scope of grant award or review "be based on ample data, and as possible, pilot testing, given the potential for unintended consequences for any system wide changes."

In recent years, the National Institutes of Health (NIH) has established initiatives that encourage impact assessments and examine programs or policies to support the biomedical workforce. For example, the NIH Common Fund funded a Coordination and Evaluation Center (CEC) to undertake longitudinal, cross-institution assessments of diversity programs such as the National Research Mentoring Network (NRMN) and the Building Infrastructure Leading to Diversity (BUILD) initiative (Estrada et al., 2016; National Academy of Sciences et al., 2011). NIH has also undertaken comprehensive evaluations of the Director's New Innovator Award (DP2) (Tinkle et al., 2016), the Director's Pioneer Award (DP1), mentored career awards, and the Institutional Research and Academic Career Development Award (IRACDA) program (K12), among others. In some cases, NIH has undertaken experimental designs to test the effect of policy changes, as is currently being done to examine anonymized peer review and implicit bias modules. For example, the NIH Scientific Workforce Diversity Office has launched an anonymized review to examine biases in peer review. That office is also assessing the efficacy of implicit bias modules and investments in research on workforce diversity. Assessments are also planned for other pilot projects for career development and mentoring, notably the Broadening Experiences in Scientific Training (BEST) program. In addition, the NIH Next Generation Researchers Initiative will be accompanied by a new effort to "encourage independent analyses of metrics that can be used to assess the impact of the NIH portfolio."

Too often, however, there is an absence of published, evidence-based studies that demonstrate the effectiveness of potential reforms on the issues that will affect the next generation of investigators. Even within NIH some successful experiments have not been considered for broader implementation, because no formal mechanism for "registering" experiments and sharing analyses exists.

This is not to say that all attempts to improve the system are equally amenable to experimentation, and if every policy change were held to the scientific method, improvements would be slow in coming. Even so, the shortage of experimentation, analyses, and sharing slows the development of much needed changes in policy that will break down the barriers confronting today's young scientists and those of future generations.

These evidence-based studies cannot be expected to emerge on their own; their conduct will require institutions, norms, and conditions that are conducive to innovation and experimentation. Fortunately, much of the institutional bedrock for such an approach already exists in the form of the embedded research capacity of our nation's graduate research programs and in the individual NIH ICs. In the recommendations that follow, the committee proposes to harness these institutions to serve as "policy laboratories" whose experiences can be used to benefit the next generation of researchers.

Recommendation 6.1
Congress and the National Institutes of Health should promote innovative pilot projects on the part of research institutions and other stakeholders that seek to improve and accelerate transitions into independent careers. A Next Generation Researcher Innovation Fund should be created to support these experimental projects.

Universities and other research institutions have been slow to adopt systemic change in how they train and support the next generation of researchers for several reasons, including a paucity of evidence that the recommended reforms of the past are effective and workable and the absence of ready resources to experiment with innovative approaches to the operation of the research enterprise. NIH has recognized the need to step in and support experimentation at the institutional level in certain areas. The BEST program, for example, supports 17 universities across the country to implement career development programs to improve access to a range of biomedical career options. The NRMN seeks to fund, implement, and evaluate innovative university approaches to research training and mentoring practices for individuals from diverse backgrounds.

These programs are laudable, but integration of sustained change into the biomedical research enterprise requires a more consistent effort to support regular experimentation and innovation that consider the full range of barriers affecting the next generation of researchers. Therefore, the committee recommends a new pilot program, perhaps run through the NIH Common Fund, to support novel experiments to improve the training and research landscape for the next generation of investigators as they seek to transition into independent research careers. The Biomedical Research Enterprise Council (BREC) described in Recommendation 3.1 could serve as a repository for all experiments proposed in Recommendations 6.1 and 6.2 (below). This pilot program could support approaches to, for example, increase the diversity of new faculty, improve support for staff scientists, and accelerate transitions to research positions in various sectors, such as academia, industry, or government. Proposals for pilot projects would be subject to NIH peer review and would address issues within or overlapping with the province of this report. The proposed experiments should be designed to include rigorous assessment, and those receiving funding under this program should be required to make results widely available at timely intervals, given that the final outcomes will take years to assess. In addition, institutions should be invited to make joint proposals or assemble consortia to submit a single proposal so that the pilots can proceed at multiple institutions where appropriate. One model for such a pilot program could be the Burroughs Wellcome Fund's Physician-

Scientist Institutional Program,[2] which provides awards of $500,000 per year over 5 years to create innovative programs to increase opportunities for physician-scientists to pursue careers in research, with careful evaluations of the funded programs.

Consistent with the need for broader stakeholder ownership of the biomedical research system, the experiments proposed in Recommendations 6.1 and 6.2 could be financed through a cost-sharing arrangement that includes NIH, universities, and industry. This approach creates incentives for stakeholders to mount programs that assist in reorienting the system, rather than the present tradition of focusing much of the responsibility for new policy reform on the shoulders of NIH. Ideally, applicants would be required to identify at least partially matching funds to ensure their commitment to the enterprise and to strengthen the impact of any initiatives designed to improve the biomedical research system.

Recommendation 6.2
The National Institutes of Health should enhance the use of its Institutes and Centers as vehicles to pilot new mechanisms designed to support the independence of early-career researchers and thereby strengthen its capacity for innovation more broadly. The Biomedical Research Enterprise Council proposed in Recommendation 3.1 should monitor and evaluate those efforts.

At NIH, policy reform involving the next generation of researchers tends to follow two broad approaches. In the first approach, a single Institute or Center develops an initiative that meet the needs of its research mission, which may later be adopted by other Institutes. For example, the National Cancer Institute (NCI)'s Research Specialist Award is designed to encourage the development of stable career opportunities for exceptional scientists who want to pursue research within the context of an existing cancer research program, but not serve as independent investigators. Another example is the National Institute of General Medical Sciences (NIGMS)'s recent decision to support early-career investigators through the Maximizing Investigators' Research Award (MIRA). Created to support established investigators, MIRA was recently expanded to include early-stage investigators and awards money to the investigator instead of a specific project, thus providing more flexibility to pursue new ideas and opportunities as they arise.[3]

The second approach to developing new policies emerges out of the NIH Office of the Director and takes several forms:

- General policies for the ICs for the administration of their grant programs, such as the early-stage and early established investigator policies through

---

[2] See https://www.bwfund.org/grant-programs/biomedical-sciences/physician-scientist-institutional-program (accessed December 6, 2017).

[3] See https://grants.nih.gov/grants/guide/pa-files/PAR-17-190.html (accessed December 6, 2017).

which the Office of the Director issued a general set of expectations for supporting certain early-career investigators;
- Parent announcements for specific grant programs that provide individual Institutes with discretion to decide the extent of their participation, such as the Pathway to Independence (K99/R00) award introduced more than a decade ago to support a timely transition from a mentored postdoctoral research position to a stable independent research position; or
- New funding programs, generally out of the Common Fund, such as the Director's New Innovator (DP2) and Early Independence Awards (DP5).

Less common is an approach that integrates these two approaches for policy change. Although programs emerge from individual institutes and centers (ICs), as well as from the NIH Office of the Director, no central and independent mechanism is charged with evaluating the performance of these experiments, and, where successful, promoting their adoption across other NIH ICs and the broader biomedical research community. An integrated approach would use the dynamic and decentralized structure of NIH ICs as natural sites for policy experimentation regarding the multi-dimensional challenges confronting young investigators. NIH should champion the rapid adoption (and tailoring, as appropriate) by all ICs of experiments proven successful through rigorous evaluation. Conversely, when evaluation provides evidence that a policy is ineffective or counterproductive, the practice or policy should be abandoned.

REFERENCES

Estrada, M., M. Burnett, A. G. Campbell, P. B. Campbell, W. F. Denetclaw, C. G. Gutiérrez, S. Hurtado, G. H. John, J. Matsui, R. McGee, C. M. Okpodu, T. J. Robinson, M. F. Summers, M. Werner-Washburne, and M. Zavala. 2016. Improving underrepresented minority student persistence in STEM. *CBE Life Sciences Education* 15(3):es5.

National Academy of Sciences, National Academy of Engineering, and Institute of Medicine. 2011. *Expanding underrepresented minority participation: America's science and technology talent at the crossroads*. Washington, DC: The National Academies Press.

Tinkle, S. S., J. C. Mary, J. E. Snavely, C. A. Pomeroy-Carter, and C. K. Tokita. 2016. *An outcome evaluation of the National Institutes of Health Director's New Innovator Award program for fiscal years 2007–2009*. Washington, DC: IDA Science & Technology Policy Institute.

7

Final Thoughts and Summary of Recommendations by Actor

The U.S. biomedical[1] research enterprise has been one of the most productive segments of the U.S. economy since the second half of the 20th century. It has been responsible for generating a wealth of knowledge about the very workings of life, producing groundbreaking medical advances, and creating thousands of new companies and tens of thousands of well-paying jobs. It has also served as a model of how multiple stakeholders, working both independently and collaboratively, can make and turn fundamental discoveries into products and economic activity that benefit many areas of modern society. Yet, as with any successful complex enterprise, sustained success — and the benefits accrued to society — requires a constant infusion of talented individuals who receive support from the enterprise as they generate the next wave of discoveries and innovations.

However, as this report and others preceding it have stated, there is substantial room for improvement when it comes to nurturing, supporting, and, in some cases, valuing that next generation of young scientists. Indeed, the U.S. biomedical enterprise is in danger of at best underutilizing and at worst losing a significant number of its brightest young scientific minds because of significant structural and cultural problems. However, stakeholders in the U.S. biomedical research enterprise, working independently and collaboratively, could implement solutions to these problems in relatively short order. Through its recommendations in this report, the committee has enumerated what it believes to be the most important of those solutions.

---

[1] In this report, "biomedical" refers to the full range of biological, biomedical, behavioral, and health sciences supported by the National Institutes of Health.

Although most of the committee's recommendations are directed at the National Institutes of Health (NIH), given its outsized role in funding biomedical research and training, they are not intended for NIH to implement by itself. In fact, of all stakeholders, NIH has been the most attentive and responsive to the issues facing emerging investigators as they strive for independent research careers. Now, it is time for the remaining stakeholders—universities and other research institutions, principal investigators, professional societies, philanthropic organizations, Congress and the nation's biomedical research funding agencies, and industry—to be equally involved in creating an environment that enables the nation's young investigators to thrive and push the frontiers of knowledge, generate enumerable benefits to our society, and provide the intellect and energy needed to keep the biomedical research enterprise strong and vibrant.

To clarify the obligations of many, though certainly not all, stakeholders to address the challenges facing young biomedical researchers, the following sections parse by stakeholder the committee's recommendations. While recommendations are assigned to a stakeholder, their implementation will often require collaborative efforts by several or all stakeholders.

THE RECOMMENDATIONS—BY STAKEHOLDER

Congress should

- Establish a Biomedical Research Enterprise Council (BREC) to address ongoing challenges confronting the Next Generation of Biomedical Researchers. The BREC would exercise ongoing collective guardianship of the biomedical enterprise function as a forum for sustained coordination, consultation, problem-solving, and assessment of progress toward implementation of the recommendations put forth in this report.
- Consider increasing the NIH budget, specifically to implement the recommendations in this report and to sustain NIH's recently announced Next Generation Researchers Initiative.
- Revise the Small Business Innovation Research (SBIR)/Small Business Technology Transfer (STTR) program to create a novel ecosystem that fosters entrepreneurship for next generation biomedical scientists, facilitates women and minority-owned entrepreneurship, and supports fulfillment of NIH's mission across the private sector.
- Extend or establish an employment tax credit to research and development (R&D) firms for hiring recently minted Ph.D.'s, M.D.'s, and M.D.-Ph.D.'s and make the credit higher for small- to medium-sized R&D firms and firms that recruit into R&D activity for the first time.
- Promote innovative pilot projects on the part of research institutions and other stakeholders that seek to improve and accelerate transitions into

independent careers. A Next Generation Researcher Innovation Fund should be created to support these experimental projects.

The National Science Foundation should

- Develop and implement a plan to improve sector-wide data collection and analysis in a manner that is easily accessible by policymakers and that integrates data from numerous other sources.
- Work expeditiously to link the Survey of Doctorate Recipients and the Survey of Earned Doctorates to U.S. Census data, and then make those linked data, under strict confidentiality protocols, available to qualified researchers at Federal Statistical Research Data Centers to understand better the biomedical workforce.

The National Institutes of Health should

- Phase-in policies that require the collection and publication of data on outcomes and demographics of biomedical pre- and postdoctoral researchers, using common standards and definitions, as a prerequisite for further funding to incentivize compliance.
- Require the inclusion of an institutional training and mentoring plan as a component of the "Resources and Environment" section of grant applications.
- Require principal investigators (PIs) to provide a postdoctoral training and mentoring plan in all grant proposals that will support postdoctoral researchers and to update those plans in progress reports.
- Increase the Ruth L. Kirschstein National Research Service Award (NRSA) starting salary for new postdoctoral researchers to $52,700 (in 2018 dollars), with annual increases for inflation and for cost-of-living tied to the Personal Consumption Expenditure Index.
- Expand awards or create new competitive awards to support postdoctoral researchers' advancement toward an independent research career. By July 2023, there should be a 5-fold increase in the number of individual research fellowship awards (F-type) and career development (K-type) awards for postdoctoral researchers granted. This goal should be achieved incrementally and steadily during this period. The indirect recovery cost rate earned by K-type and training awards should be increased to 16 percent.
- Phase in a cap (3 years suggested) on salary support for all postdoctoral researchers funded by NIH research grants and multi-project grants. This phase in should occur only after a robust pilot study (or studies) of sufficient size and duration to assess the feasibility of this policy and the opportunities it provides has been undertaken.

- Work with Congress to revise the SBIR/STTR program to create a novel ecosystem that fosters entrepreneurship for next generation biomedical scientists, supports women and minority-owned entrepreneurship, and facilitates fulfillment of NIH's mission across the private sector.
- Increase the number of NIH Director's New Innovator Awards (DP2), and similar programs funded by individual NIH Institutes and Centers, to promote innovative research with high potential for groundbreaking discoveries.
- Ensure that the duration of all R01 research grants supporting early-stage investigators (ESIs) is no less than 5 years to enable the establishment of resilient and independent research programs. NIH Institutes and Centers should experiment with further extending the duration of R01 awards for ESIs.
- Retain the ESI status for individuals who participate in multi-PI submissions prior to receiving their own R01 grants, unless serving as a co-PI on a funded multi-PI award provides them with R01-equivalent funds for their own research, to avoid dis-incentivizing research collaboration.
- Expand the Pathways to Independence (K99/R00) award but prioritize fostering independence through career development. The award should require development of an innovative and independent research project that is conceived of and executed by the applicant. The award should not represent additional or new training.
- Continue to improve the peer-review process to optimize the evaluation of applications submitted by early-stage and early experienced investigators in the Next Generation Researchers Initiative. This is of special importance for investigators from underrepresented groups.
- Revise the biosketch requirement to focus peer review on recent contributions and accomplishments and continue to test effective practices for reducing the effects of implicit bias and for increasing the diversity of reviewers.
- Develop mechanisms to increase the number of individuals in staff scientist positions to provide more stable, non-faculty research opportunities for the next generation of researchers.
- Require an institutional diversity and inclusion plan as a part of the Institutional Resources component of research grants to promote diversity and inclusion at the junior faculty level.
- Allocate funds from the Next Generation Researchers Initiative to expand the number of Research Supplements to Promote Diversity in Health-Related Research (PA-16-288). Award these supplements to underrepresented minority ESIs and investigators who have not received a prior research project grant and seek to collaborate with funded investigators on new but related research projects.

- Offer the Loan Repayment Programs to all individuals pursuing biomedical physician-scientist researcher careers, regardless of their research area or clinical specialty, and increase the amount of loan forgiveness to reflect the debt burden of current medical trainees.
- Continue implementation of the recommendations set forth in the 2014 NIH *Physician-Scientist Workforce Working Group Report*, and test new strategies and expand effective approaches to increase the pool of early-stage physician-scientists.
- Promote innovative pilot projects of research institutions and other stakeholders that seek to improve and accelerate transitions into independent careers. Create a Next Generation Researcher Innovation Fund to support these experimental projects.
- Enhance the use of Institutes and Centers as vehicles to pilot new mechanisms designed to support the independence of early-career researchers and thereby strengthen NIH capacity for innovation more broadly. Monitor and evaluate these pilots through the Biomedical Research Enterprise Council proposed above.

Biomedical research institutions should

- Promote, document, and disseminate existing and planned efforts, both independent and collaborative, to reduce the barriers to recruiting and retaining diverse researchers for pre- and postdoctoral positions and the initial stages of research independence.
- Collect, analyze, and disseminate comprehensive data on outcomes, demographics, and career aspirations of biomedical pre- and postdoctoral researchers using common standards and definitions as developed in concert with NIH.
- Provide evidence to NIH of formal training of faculty mentors of postdoctoral trainees.
- Adjust the base postdoctoral salary annually to match the corresponding NRSA rate, with increases based on local cost-of-living, and harmonize benefits for all postdoctoral scholars regardless of their support mechanism.
- Levy a fee of at least $1,000 per year for each postdoctoral fellow supported on all biomedical research grants. These fees should be used to support effective training and professional development programs for postdoctoral researchers, as well as effective training of mentors. The use of the fees should be reported publicly.
- Identify or provide an institutional ombudsperson to resolve fairly and expeditiously conflicts and concerns between principal investigators and postdoctoral researchers related to the training experience.
- Limit postdoctoral training to 5 years, after which postdoctoral researchers continuing in the same laboratory should be shifted to employment as a staff

scientist with an increase in salary and benefits appropriate for a permanent staff member.
- Develop mechanisms to increase the number of individuals in staff scientist positions to provide more stable, non-faculty research opportunities for the next generation of researchers.
- Experiment with creating career tracks for staff scientists with clearly defined review and promotion processes, as well as opportunities for professional development.
- `Provide individuals in the staff scientist track with salaries and benefits commensurate with their experiences and responsibilities.

Principal investigators should

- Provide every postdoctoral researcher with a high-quality training experience that prepares them for a successful research career.
- Receive formal training from their research institutions on mentoring postdoctoral trainees.
- Provide a postdoctoral training and mentoring plan in all grant proposals and updates of those plans in all progress reports to NIH if funded.
- Provide a diversity and inclusion plan in all grant proposals and updates of those plans in all progress reports to NIH if funded.

A

Definitions Used in the Report

Biomedical—The full range of biological, biomedical, behavioral, and health sciences supported by the National Institutes of Health.

Early-Stage Investigator (ESI)—A Program Director/Principal Investigator (PD/PI) who has completed their terminal research degree or post-graduate clinical training, whichever date is later, within the past 10 years and who has not previously competed successfully as PD/PI for a substantial NIH independent research award.[1] This report also refers to ESIs as early-career investigators.

Early Established Investigator (EEI)—A PD/PI who is within 10 years of receiving their first substantial, independent competing NIH R01 equivalent research award as an ESI.[2]

Independent Researcher—An individual who enjoys independence of thought—the freedom to define the problem of interest and/or to choose or develop the best strategies and approaches to address that problem. Under this definition, an independent scientist may work alone, as the intellectual leader of a research group, or as a member of a consortium of investigators each contributing distinct expertise. Specifically, we do not intend "independence" to mean necessarily "isolated" or "solitary," or to imply "self-sustaining" or "separately funded."

---

[1] See https://grants.nih.gov/policy/early-investigators/index.htm (accessed February 15, 2018).
[2] See https://grants.nih.gov/policy/early-investigators/index.htm (accessed February 15, 2018).

Postdoctoral Researcher—An individual in a period of mentored transition to independence, providing (1) increasing intellectual control of scientific direction and (2) professional development in skills necessary to lead a research project.

Underrepresented Minorities (URM)—Three racial or ethnic minority groups (blacks, Hispanics, and American Indians or Native Alaskans) whose representation in science and engineering education or employment is smaller than their representation in the U.S. population.[3]

---

[3] NSF. Women, Minorities, and Persons with Disabilities in Science and Engineering 2017. https://www.nsf.gov/statistics/2017/nsf17310/digest/glossary-and-key-to-acronyms/ (accessed February 7, 2018).

B

Responses to Recommendations in Previous Reports on Biomedical and Behavioral Researchers

August 2017

Prepared by Yasmeen Hussain, Ph.D., and Amanda Field, Ph.D., for the Committee on the Next Generation Researchers Initiative[1]

The following discussion and conclusions were checked for accuracy by the National Institutes of Health.

The Committee on the Next Generation Researchers Initiative is not the first to examine the challenges young investigators face in starting independent research careers. Indeed, over the past few decades, a number of groups have issued high-profile reports examining concerns about the biomedical and behavioral research enterprise and the investigators trained to carry out that research. These reports each contained recommendations that targeted various institutions, career stages, and scientific research organizations, and all were aimed at securing and supporting our nation's biomedical and behavioral research scientists.

The committee recognized early in its work that while a number of previous recommendations have been offered to tackle these concerns, only some of those recommendations actually had seen progress in the ensuing years. This led the committee, early in its deliberations, to pose a series of questions: Which of the previous recommendations had been addressed, and which had not? Of those that had been addressed, had interventions addressed the challenges confronting the biomedical workforce, or had they produced unintended consequences? Answering these questions was instrumental in informing the work of the committee.

---

[1] The discussion and conclusions in this paper were checked for accuracy by the National Institutes of Health. This paper is not an official report of the National Academies of Sciences, Engineering, and Medicine. Opinions and statements included in this material are solely those of the individual authors and do not necessarily represent the views of the committee or the National Academies.

The committee collected relevant recommendations from the National Academies of Sciences, Engineering, and Medicine reports dating back to 2005, as well as three National Institutes of Health (NIH) working group reports and a 2015 report from the Federation of American Societies for Experimental Biology (FASEB):

- *Bridges to Independence: Fostering the Independence of New Investigators in Biomedical Research* (2005). National Research Council of the National Academies.
- *Research Training in the Biomedical, Behavioral and Clinical Research Sciences* (2011). National Research Council of the National Academies.
- *Biomedical Research Workforce Working Group Report* (2012). National Institutes of Health.
- *Report of the Advisory Committee to the Director Working Group on Diversity in the Biomedical Research Workforce* (2012). National Institutes of Health.
- *Physician-Scientist Workforce Working Group Report* (2014). National Institutes of Health.
- *The Postdoctoral Experience Revisited* (2014). National Academy of Sciences, National Academy of Engineering, and Institute of Medicine of the National Academies.
- *Sustaining Discovery in Biological and Medical Sciences: A Framework for Discussion* (2015). Federation of American Societies for Experimental Biology.

The recommendations from these reports that addressed concerns facing early-career investigators fell into seven target areas: postdoctoral practices, diversity in the research workforce, data collection, early career support, faculty support, staff scientist support, and grant review. This paper explores the recommendations in each of these areas in turn.

1. RECOMMENDATIONS ON POSTDOCTORAL PRACTICES

Postdoctoral training has become a nearly de facto requirement for an independent research career in the biomedical and behavioral sciences in the United States. While most U.S.-trained biomedical Ph.D.'s spend fewer than 5 years in postdoctoral training, significant numbers remain in postdoctoral positions between 5 and 8 years.[2] The postdoctoral experience is nominally considered an opportunity to build skills and experiences to prepare for research independence. According to the 2014 *Postdoctoral Experience Revisited* report, postdoctoral re-

---

[2] See https://acd.od.nih.gov/documents/reports/Biomedical_research_wgreport.pdf, p. 21; S. Kahn and D. K. Ginther, The impact of postdoctoral training on early careers in biomedicine, *Nat Bio*, 2017 Jan, 35(1), 90-94.

searchers should be receiving advanced training in research, and at the end of the appointment, the postdoctoral researcher should transition to a permanent position accompanied by a change in job duties and compensation. However, prior reports have called out the postdoctoral research stage as a "holding pattern" for young scientists.[3] As such, the reports we examined made several recommendations germane to postdoctoral researchers.

> **1.1 NIH should enforce a 5-year limit on the use of any funding mechanism to support postdoctoral researchers with the nature of the position, including responsibilities and benefits, changing for those researchers who transition to staff scientist positions after 5 years (normal duration should be 3 years).**
> *Bridges to Independence (2005)*
> *The Postdoctoral Experience Revisited (2014)*

While there is no explicit general action by NIH beyond guidance for all supported postdoctoral researchers,[4] NIH has instituted time limits for some of its training programs. For example, there is a statutory and regulatory limit on the duration of support for postdoctoral researchers supported by a National Research Service Award (NRSA). The NRSA legislation specifies that total support for postdoctoral researchers may not exceed 3 years, but waivers are allowed for good cause.[5] NIH enforces this limit, with any period of additional support on NRSA training grants or fellowships requiring approval from the awarding institute that supports the training grant or fellowship.[6] In 2014, NIH reduced the eligibility for Pathway to Independence Award Program (K99/R00) applications from 5 years to no more than 4 years of postdoctoral research experience at the time of the initial application or subsequent resubmission. The intent was to further encourage early transition to independence.[7,8]

Although NIH has taken some steps to impose time limits for postdoctoral appointments, postdoctoral researchers on research grants are almost always employees of their institutions and subject to employment policies at that institution. NIH is limited in its ability to independently modify or require specific changes in employment practices at grantee institutions. That being said, NIH went on record in 2001 supporting a 5-year limit on postdoctoral training experiences from any

---

[3] *Trends in the Early Careers of Life Scientists* (1998); *Bridges to Independence* (2005).
[4] See https://grants.nih.gov/grants/guide/notice-files/NOT-OD-01-027.html (accessed December 11, 2017).
[5] 42 USC 288(b)(4), as implemented by 42 CFR §§ 66.106(e) and 66.205(b).
[6] See https://www.law.cornell.edu/uscode/text/42/288 (accessed December 11, 2017).
[7] See https://grants.nih.gov/grants/guide/pa-files/PA-14-042.html (accessed December 11, 2017).
[8] See https://nexus.od.nih.gov/all/2013/05/16/more-information-on-the-k99r00-awards/ (accessed December 11, 2017).

source of federal dollars.[9] Some institutions have established their own time limits on postdoctoral appointments. In 2008, for example, New York University School of Medicine imposed a 5-year limit on postdoctoral length, including time spent in previous postdoctoral experiences. The University of California system and University of North Carolina have reportedly implemented less-strict limits.[10]

> **1.2 The title of "postdoctoral researcher" should only be applied to those people receiving advanced training in research. Funding agencies should have a consistent designation for "postdoctoral researchers" and require evidence of advanced research training. Institutions should create professional positions for individuals who are conducting research but who are not receiving training, such as permanent staff scientists.**
> *The Postdoctoral Experience Revisited (2014)*

There has been no known uniform action on the titles of postdoctoral researchers supported by research project grants (RPGs). Most universities have policy guidance stipulating that postdoctoral researchers should receive training. Nevertheless, it is not clear whether universities instituted these policies before or after the report's recommendations, and it is not clear whether these policies reflect the extent of training that postdoctoral researchers receive.[11,12]

However, all postdoctoral researchers supported by NIH NRSA funds via training grants or fellowships are said to be in training. For individuals supported on research grants, the grantee institutions assign the title, and institutions or principal investigators (PIs) assign the duties of the postdoctoral researcher.[13]

> **1.3 NIH, academic institutions, and research institutions should increase training and mentoring of postdoctoral researchers.**
> *Bridges to Independence (2005)*
> *The Postdoctoral Experience Revisited (2014)*

> **Structured training experience for postdoctoral researchers should be provided by requiring individual development plans (IDPs) for all NIH-supported postdoctoral researchers.**
> *Biomedical Research Workforce Working Group Report (2012)*

---

[9] See https://grants.nih.gov/grants/guide/notice-files/NOT-OD-01-027.html (accessed December 11, 2017).

[10] See http://www.nature.com/news/the-future-of-the-postdoc-1.17253 (accessed December 11, 2017).

[11] See http://www.columbia.edu/cu/vpaa/handbook/research.html (accessed December 11, 2017).

[12] See http://www.hr.virginia.edu/hr-for-you/professional-research-staff/ (accessed December 11, 2017).

[13] See https://grants.nih.gov/grants/guide/pa-files/PA-16-307.html (accessed December 11, 2017).

Some NIH programs and policies have aimed to increase training experiences for postdoctoral researchers and graduate students. In 2013, NIH encouraged institutions to develop and use IDPs for postdoctoral researchers and graduate students. In 2014, NIH issued a notice to indicate that NIH annual progress reports received on or after October 1, 2014, must include a section describing how IDPs are used to identify and promote the career goals of graduate students and postdoctoral researchers associated with NIH awards. This is required for research project grants supporting graduate students and postdoctoral researchers and for all T, F, K, R25, D43, and other awards or award components designed to provide training and professional development opportunities for graduate students and postdoctoral researchers.[14,15] NIH also launched the K99/R00 Pathway to Independence awards in 2006 in response to the *Bridges to Independence* report and specified a mentoring component and training plan relating to the candidate's career goals.[16]

1.4 NIH should increase the proportion of postdoctoral researchers supported by training grants and fellowships.
Bridges to Independence (2005)
Biomedical Research Workforce Working Group Report (2012)

The number of T32 and F32 postdoctoral training grants and fellowships has remained relatively constant since these recommendations were made (see section 1.6 below for more detail). In 2013, following the Biomedical Research Workforce Report review, NIH declared its intention to increase support for the K99/R00 Pathway to Independence awards, aiming for a 30 percent success rate compared to the 23 percent success rate in 2012 (Figure B-1).

Outside of NIH, some private foundations have developed new postdoctoral fellowships. For example, the Simons Foundation responded to the NIH report by developing its Bridge to Independence Award to invest in and support early investigators in autism research.[17] Similarly, the Howard Hughes Medical Institute initiated the Hanna Gray Fellowship Program in 2016 to support researchers for a minimum of 2 and a maximum of 4 years of postdoctoral training and up to 4 years of a tenure-track faculty position at a U.S. institution with a doctoral-level graduate program in the fellow's field of interest.[18] Other privately funded postdoctoral research award programs include the Damon Runyon Fellowship

---

[14] See https://biomedicalresearchworkforce.nih.gov/improve.htm (accessed December 11, 2017).

[15] See https://grants.nih.gov/grants/guide/notice-files/NOT-OD-14-113.html (accessed December 11, 2017).

[16] See https://www.nih.gov/news-events/news-releases/nih-announces-program-foster-independence-new-investigators, initial funding opportunity announcement: https://grants.nih.gov/grants/guide/pa-files/PA-07-297.html (accessed December 11, 2017).

[17] See https://www.simonsfoundation.org/funding/funding-opportunities/autism-research-initiative-sfari/bridge-to-independence-award-request-for-applications/ (accessed December 11, 2017).

[18] See https://www.hhmi.org/news/hhmi-launches-new-program-early-career-scientists (accessed December 11, 2017).

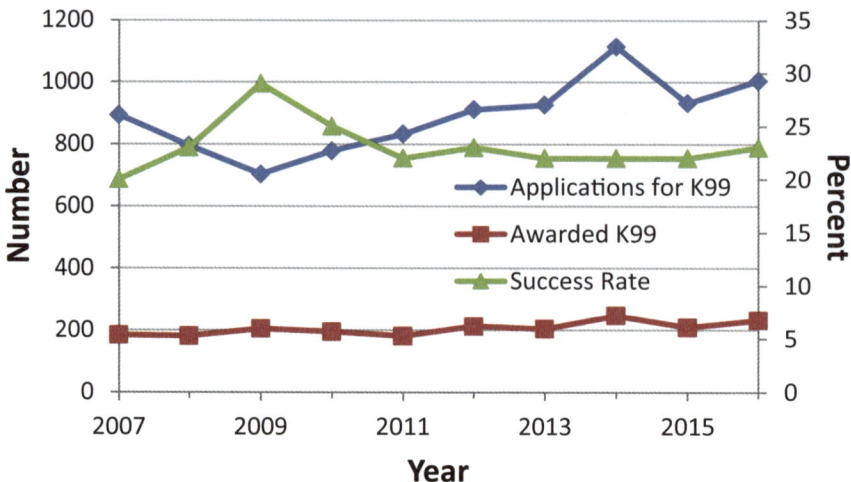

FIGURE B-1 Trends in the K99 research career development award: Competing applications and awards between 2007 and 2016.
SOURCE: NIH IMPAC, Success Rate File.

Award,[19] the American Association for Cancer Research Postdoctoral and Clinical Research Fellow Grants,[20] and the American Heart Association Postdoctoral Fellowship.[21]

The recommendation to increase the proportion of postdoctoral researchers supported by training grants and fellowships has received some resistance from the research community. For example, the Association of Medical and Graduate Departments of Biochemistry (AMGDB) published a response on behalf of its leaders through the American Society for Biochemistry and Molecular Biology (ASBMB) detailing its opposition to the Biomedical Research Workforce report recommendation.[22] In its response, the AMGDB leaders opposed increasing the number of postdoctoral fellows supported through training grants, asserting that postdoctoral salary support though R01 grants is a historically effective mechanism to easily and efficiently accommodate productivity and achievement.

---

[19] See https://www.damonrunyon.org/for-scientists/application-guidelines/fellowship (accessed December 11, 2017).

[20] See http://www.aacr.org/FUNDING/PAGES/POSTDOCTORAL-AND-CLINICAL-RESEARCH-FELLOW-GRANT-RECIPIENTS___DFCBB5.ASPX#.WYH6A1GQzRZ (accessed December 11, 2017).

[21] See http://professional.heart.org/professional/ResearchPrograms/ApplicationInformation/UCM_443314_Postdoctoral-Fellowship.jsp (accessed December 11, 2017).

[22] See http://www.asbmb.org/asbmbtoday/201409/Education/ (accessed December 11, 2017).

APPENDIX B 115

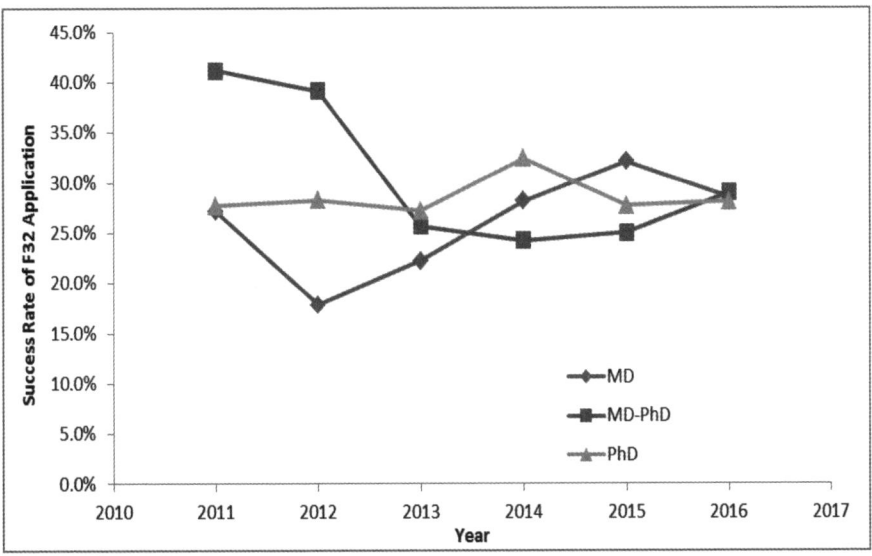

FIGURE B-2 Trends in F32 awards: The success rate for F32 applications by degree between 2011 and 2016.
SOURCE: NIH IMPAC, Success Rate File.

1.5 NIH should shift the balance in NRSA postdoctoral training for physicians so that greater proportions are supported through individual fellowships, rather than institutional training grants.
Physician-Scientist Workforce Working Group Report (2014)

Thus far, there is no known action addressing this recommendation.

Physician-scientists with professional health degrees are eligible to apply for individual postdoctoral fellowships known as F32 awards and receive special consideration under NRSA legislation if they agree to undertake a minimum of 2 years of biomedical research.[23,24,25] Available data indicate that a majority of applicants and awardees for postdoctoral fellowships hold a Ph.D., but the success rate for those physician-scientists who apply is similar to that of Ph.D.-only applicants (Figure B-2). In 2016, the success rate for F32 applicants with the following degrees was 28.1 percent for Ph.D.'s, 28.6 percent for M.D.'s, and

---

[23] See https://grants.nih.gov/grants/guide/pa-files/PA-16-307.html (accessed December 11, 2017).
[24] See https://www.law.cornell.edu/uscode/text/42/288 (accessed December 11, 2017).
[25] See https://grants.nih.gov/grants/policy/nihgps_2012/nihgps_ch11.htm (accessed December 11, 2017).

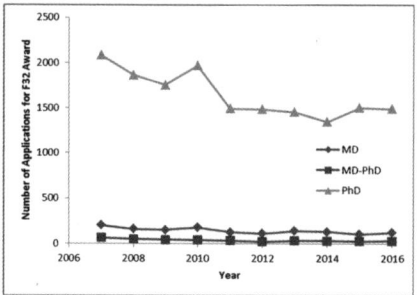
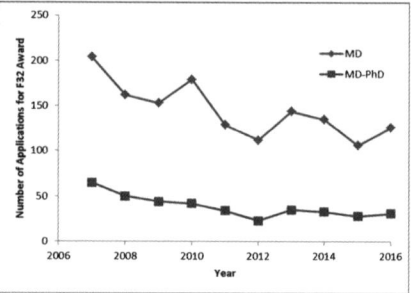
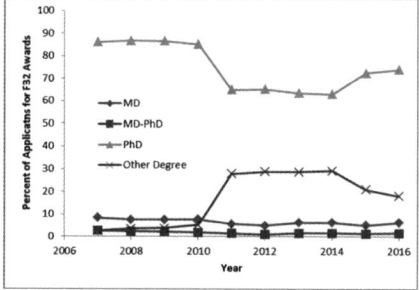

FIGURE B-3 Trends in F32 applications: Numbers of competing applications (top left: all applicants; top right: medical degree-holding applicants only) and percent of applicants with particular degrees (bottom: all applicants) between 2007 and 2016.
SOURCE: NIH IMPAC, Success Rate File.

29 percent for M.D.-Ph.D.'s.[26] Over the past decade, the number of applications for individual postdoctoral fellowships from physician-scientists has declined, as has the number from applicants with Ph.D. degrees (Figure B-3). At the same time, NIH has offered opportunities for physician-scientist training through the Clinical Translational Science Awards (CTSA), established in 2006 (8 years prior to Recommendation 1-5). Nearly 300 physician-scientists a year receive support to develop their research careers through institutional career development awards associated with CTSAs.[27] Other mechanisms, such as institutional K12 awards provided by multiple Institutes and that support both physicians and basic scien-

---

[26] See https://report.nih.gov/success_rates/index.aspx, "Postdoctoral fellowships (F32s): Applications, awards, success rates, and funding, by degree of applicant" (accessed December 11, 2017).

[27] See https://report.nih.gov/success_rates/index.aspx, "Postdoctoral fellowships (F32s): Applications, awards, success rates, and funding, by degree of applicant" (accessed December 11, 2017).

tists are also available.[28] Discussions are ongoing as to the most effective ways to support postdoctoral training of physician scientists through fellowships and other mechanisms.

1.6 The total number of NRSA positions should remain at previous fiscal year levels.
Research Training in the Biomedical, Behavioral and Clinical Research Sciences (2011)

The total number of NRSA postdoctoral positions, which includes both T32 and F32 awards, has remained relatively constant since the report's release in 2011. F32 awards have remained at approximately 500 to 600 awards per year, and T32 awards, which each support varied numbers of pre- and/or postdoctoral training slots, have ranged between approximately 300 and 400 awards per year (Figures B-4 and B-5).

1.7 Institutions should better communicate career prospects to trainees and facilitate broader educational and training opportunities.
Bridges to Independence (2005)
Biomedical Research Workforce Working Group Report (2012)
Sustaining Discovery in Biological and Medical Sciences, FASEB (2015)

In 2014, prior to FASEB's release of this recommendation, NIH changed the instructions related to career preparation of individuals supported by NRSA training programs to reflect changes in career opportunities. This change occurred after similar recommendations were made in the Biomedical Workforce Working Group report to the Advisory Committee to the Director of NIH in 2012. The program announcement associated with this change specifies that trainees should receive preparation for research-related careers, as well as research-intensive careers, in various sectors, e.g., academic institutions, government agencies, for-profit businesses, and private foundations.[29] The instructions also state that training programs should make available structured career development, advising, and learning opportunities (e.g., workshops, discussions, IDPs).

In 2013, prior to the FASEB report release, NIH launched the "Strengthening the Biomedical Research Workforce" program through the Common Fund as one component of a trans-NIH strategy to enhance training opportunities for early-career scientists that would prepare them for a variety of research-related

---

[28] For example: https://grants.nih.gov/grants/guide/pa-files/PAR-16-103.html; https://grants.nih.gov/grants/guide/pa-files/PAR-16-189.html; https://grants.nih.gov/grants/guide/rfa-files/RFA-HL-17-016.html; https://grants.nih.gov/grants/guide/rfa-files/RFA-HD-17-021.html; https://grants.nih.gov/grants/guide/rfa-files/RFA-NS-17-010.html (accessed December 11, 2017).

[29] See https://grants.nih.gov/grants/guide/pa-files/PA-16-152.html (accessed December 11, 2017).

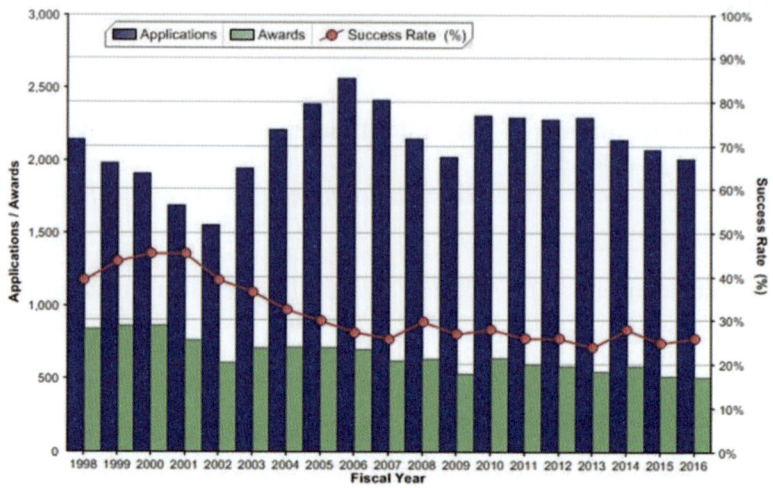
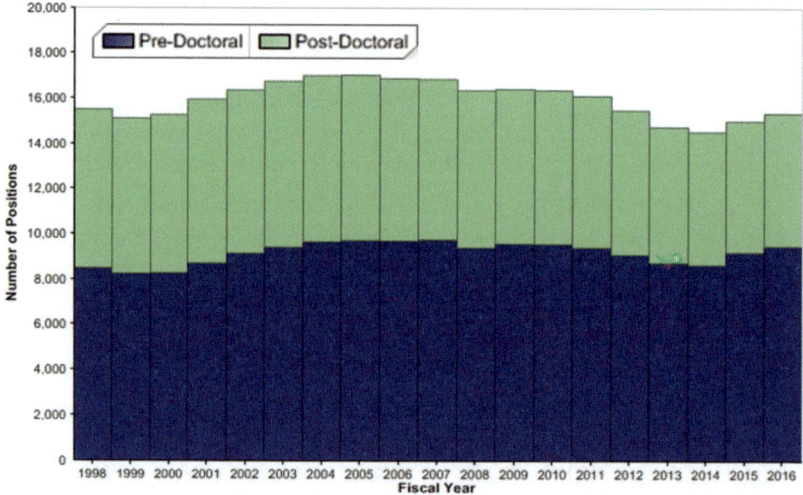

FIGURE B-4 Trends in NRSA awards: (top) Competing applications, awards, and success rates between 1998 and 2016 for F32 postdoctoral fellowships; (bottom) Awarded NRSA training and fellowship positions by pre-doctoral and postdoctoral status between 1998 and 2016.
SOURCE: (top) NIH Data Book; (bottom) NIH Correspondence.

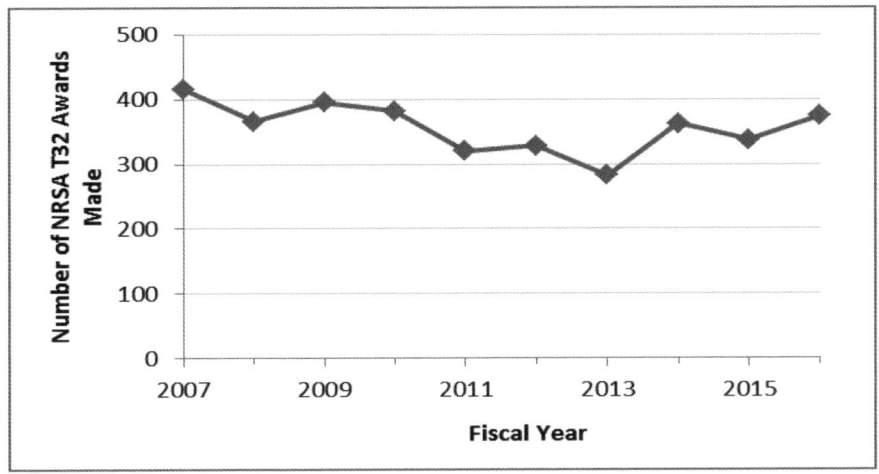

FIGURE B-5 Trends in T32 awards: Number of awards between 2007 and 2016.
SOURCE: NIH Success Rates.

career options.[30] The core component of this program is the NIH Director's Biomedical Research Workforce Innovation Award to enhance biomedical research training, more commonly called the Broadening Experiences in Scientific Training (BEST) awards. These 5-year awards are intended to support innovation in both graduate student and postdoctoral researcher training.[31] The first application cycle for BEST was in 2013. Ten awards were issued in fall 2013, and seven additional awards were made in 2014. However, the BEST program is limited to 17 institutions, and no known long-term action has been taken by NIH to continue the program because Common Fund programs are not renewable. Evaluation of the outcomes and dissemination of the best practices beyond the 17 institutions, however, is a key requirement of the current BEST program. Additionally, NIH hosted a "Best Practices Meeting" in 2017 to discuss how to disseminate best practices and lessons learned from the BEST Programs.[32]

NIH has worked with the National Academies on the University Industry Demonstration Partnership (UIDP) to identify and coordinate activities related to enhanced and more targeted career development options for both graduate students and postdoctoral researchers. One example of an activity is a November 2016 workshop that discussed approaches for improving nonacademic career information flow.[33]

---

[30] See https://commonfund.nih.gov/workforce/fundedresearch (accessed December 11, 2017).
[31] See http://www.nihbest.org/about-best/ (accessed December 11, 2017).
[32] See http://www.nihbest.org/2017best-practices-workshop/ (accessed December 11, 2017).
[33] See https://www.uidp.org/non-academic-pathways/ (accessed December 11, 2017).

Some higher education institutions are implementing programs outside of the BEST structure, such as the Biomedical Careers Initiative at Johns Hopkins,[34] to better communicate career prospects to their trainees. Other academic institutions have implemented programs to expand postdoctoral training. For example, the University of Washington instituted the Broadening the Representation of Academic Investigators in Neuroscience (BRAINS) program in 2013, funded by an R25 grant from the National Institute for Neurological Disorders and Stroke, to support professional development of researchers from underrepresented groups.[35] An evaluation of the first two cohorts indicated that participation in BRAINS yielded improved professional development confidence and activity, as well as parity in job outcomes for underrepresented minority researchers.[36] However, there is no evidence of a unified action by research-intensive universities, research institutions, and other host institutions to provide career development opportunities for postdoctoral researchers.

Some other organizations have programs that aim to address the need for career preparation for postdoctoral researchers. The National Science Foundation (NSF) piloted the Discovery Corps Fellowship Program to identify new postdoctoral and professional development models that combine research with service-oriented projects.[37] However, this program began before the release of the reports, and no known widespread action has been taken by NSF in response to this recommendation. Many professional societies, including the ASBMB, FASEB, AAMC, the American Association for the Advancement of Science (AAAS), the Council of Graduate Schools (CGS), and the Center for Biomedical Career Development, are devoting efforts to broaden career preparation for their members.

1.8 NIH should increase postdoctoral fellow stipends.
Research Training in the Biomedical, Behavioral and Clinical Research Sciences (2011)
Biomedical Research Workforce Working Group Report (2012)
The Postdoctoral Experience Revisited (2014)

While the recommended stipend levels from the three reports differ, NIH increased NRSA stipends for starting level postdoctoral trainees and fellows between FY2014 and FY2017. As of 2017, NIH postdoctoral stipend levels have reached the minimum level recommended by the *Biomedical Research Workforce* report but not the minimum recommended by the *Postdoctoral Research Experience* report. The 2017 NRSA stipends in constant 2012 dollars are at 1975 levels following a period of declining salary levels before 1998 (Figure B-6).

---

[34] See http://bci.jhmi.edu/About percent20BCI (accessed December 11, 2017).
[35] See http://depts.washington.edu/brains/program.html (accessed December 11, 2017).
[36] See http://www.lifescied.org/content/15/3/ar49.full (accessed December 11, 2017).
[37] See https://www.nsf.gov/funding/pgm_summ.jsp?pims_id=6676 (accessed December 11, 2017).

APPENDIX B

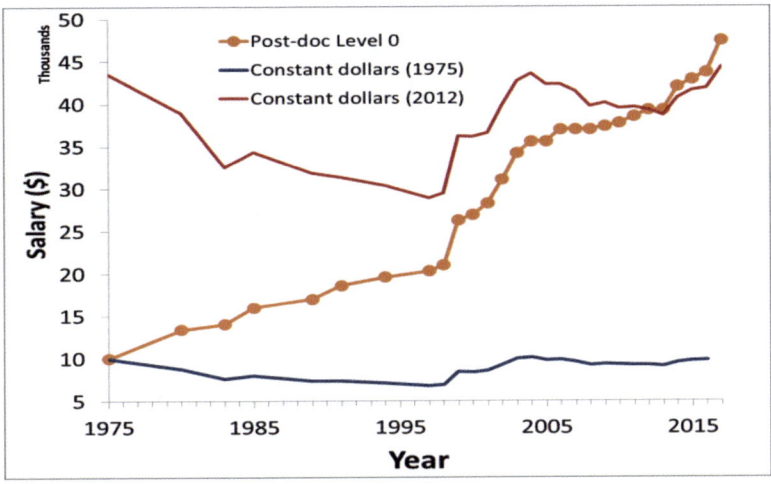

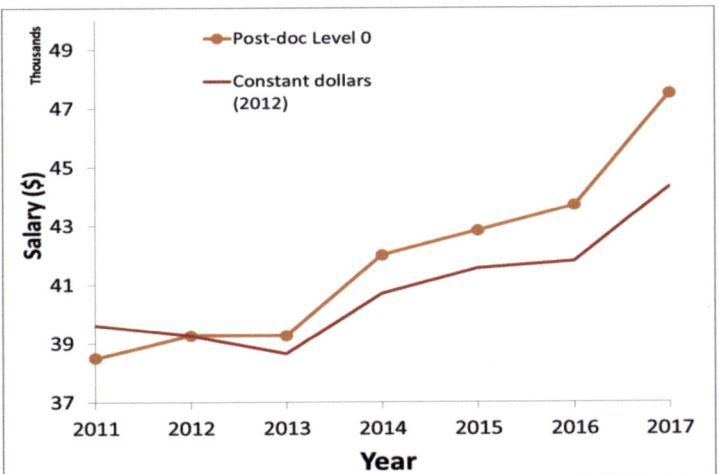

FIGURE B-6 NRSA postdoctoral salaries in nominal and constant dollars. Left: in constant 1975 and 2012 dollars since 1975; Right: in 2012 dollars since 2011.
SOURCE: NIH NRSA notices, BLS Inflation Tool for CPI adjustment.

The Department of Labor proposed a rule that updated overtime regulations by expanding eligibility under the Fair Labor Standards Act (FLSA) to employees earning a salary of less than $913 per week. However, on November 23, 2016, a United States District judge imposed an injunction, temporarily stopping the rule's enforcement nationwide, in order to have time to determine whether the Department of Labor had the authority to issue the regulation. In response to the FLSA revision, the NIH director announced that NIH will work to raise NRSA awards above the threshold,[38] and the 2017 NRSA starting postdoctoral stipend was increased to $47,484. Stipends at all other postdoctoral levels were also increased in 2017.

1.9 NIH should increase indirect cost rates on NRSA training grants and K awards.
Research Training in the Biomedical, Behavioral and Clinical Research Sciences (2011)

NIH reports that it has assessed the costs related to the NRSA program and concluded that many institutional costs normally covered by indirect cost payments can be reimbursed via tuition payments allowed under NRSA. NIH therefore has not taken any further action on this matter.

1.10 Postdoctoral researchers supported on NIH research grants should receive comparable benefits to other employees at the institution.
Biomedical Research Workforce Working Group Report (2012)

Postdoctoral researchers are often considered employees of their institution and are thus subject to institutional policies. Therefore, in direct response to this recommendation, NIH solicited input from the extramural postdoctoral community in early 2014 on benefits currently provided to postdoctoral researchers to identify opportunities to equalize benefits across various support mechanisms.[39,40] The content of the community comments is currently unknown. However, in 2015, NIH conducted a survey of institutions—50 percent responded—to understand benefits for postdoctoral researchers supported on different mechanisms. Responses to the survey indicated that many institutions provide postdoctoral researchers supported on research grants with benefits such as standard health insurance that are comparable to other employees (Figure B-7). Nevertheless, survey responses also revealed variation across institutions and funding mechanisms.[41]

In response to these survey results, the NIH Office of Extramural Research convened a working group titled "Benefits for National Research Service Award

---

[38] See http://www.huffingtonpost.com/francis-s-collins-M.D.-Ph.D./fair-pay-for-postdocs-why_b_10011066.html (accessed December 11, 2017).

[39] See https://biomedicalresearchworkforce.nih.gov/docs/Postdoc_survey_sample_letter.pdf (accessed December 11, 2017).

[40] See https://grants.nih.gov/grants/guide/notice-files/NOT-OD-13-045.html (accessed December 11, 2017).

[41] See https://nexus.od.nih.gov/all/2015/11/30/update-postdoctoral-benefit-survey/ (accessed December 11, 2017).

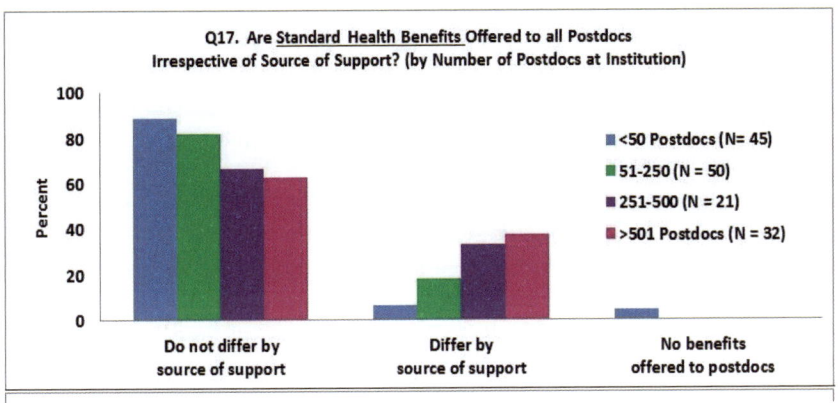

FIGURE B-7 Survey of health benefits for postdoctoral researchers.
SOURCE: NIH Survey of Institutions.

Postdoctoral Researchers" to discuss optimization of benefits provided to postdoctoral trainees and fellows supported on NRSA awards. NIH reports that the group provided recommendations to address the issue and will contribute to an implementation plan in 2017.[42] NIH also issued a notice to clarify that recipients of NRSA awards are eligible for 8 weeks of paid family leave.[43]

1.11 Provide new postdoctoral independent research awards at NIH that would complement NRSA.

Bridges to Independence (2005)

NIH established two award mechanisms that address this recommendation: the K99/R00 Pathway to Independence awards and the NIH Director's Early Independence Award (DP5). NIH launched the K99/R00 award in 2006-2007 (more details on the K99/R00 are provided in section 1-13), and NIH has awarded some 200 to 250 K99 awards annually since 2012.[44] NIH launched the DP5 award in 2011 to support investigators pursuing independent research directly after completing a terminal doctoral/research degree or clinical residency. NIH has funded approximately 10 to 16 awards annually since 2011.

Relevant NIH programs in existence prior to this recommendation include the Mentored Research Scientist Career Development Award for basic and behav-

---

[42] See https://dpcpsi.nih.gov/collaborations/committees.aspx?TID=2#14 (accessed December 11, 2017).

[43] See https://grants.nih.gov/grants/guide/notice-files/NOT-OD-16-105.html (accessed December 11, 2017).

[44] See https://www.nih.gov/news-events/news-releases/nih-announces-program-foster-independence-new-investigators (accessed December 11, 2017).

ioral scientists (K01), other K awards that support physician-scientists to pursue basic, translational (K08) or patients-oriented mentored research (K23) with a goal to transition to independence, and the Ruth L. Kirschstein Interdisciplinary Research Training Award (T90) and combined Research Education Grant (R90). The purpose of the K01 is to provide support and "protected time" (over 3, 4, or 5 years) for an intensive, supervised career development experience in the biomedical, behavioral, or clinical sciences leading to research independence.[45] There has been a growth in K01 awards from 82 in 1997 to 202 in 2016.[46] The K awards that support physician-scientists are discussed later in this document.

The T90 and R90 are institutional programs that together support comprehensive interdisciplinary research training programs, but the R90 gives support to those who do not meet qualifications for NRSA support. The T90 component supports postdoctoral researchers through institutional NRSA awards and does not provide individual independent research awards to postdoctoral researchers.[47]

1.12 The citizenship requirement for NRSAs should be modified to provide equal opportunities for non-U.S. citizens.
Bridges to Independence (2005)

To be eligible for an NRSA award, individuals must be U.S. citizens, non-citizen nationals of the United States, or lawfully admitted to the United States for permanent residence at the time of the award. This is mandated by NRSA statute 42 CFR 66.103(a); any modification would require legislative action.

There is currently no citizenship requirement for K99 applicants, but significantly more individual postdoctoral NRSA fellowships (approximately 550-650 annually) are awarded than K99s (approximately 200 annually). In addition, NRSA awards support postdoctoral researchers, while the K99/R00 supports postdoctoral researchers transitioning to independent faculty positions. However, research grants such as R01s support significantly more postdoctoral researchers than either NRSAs or K99s. Institutions make the decisions regarding hiring decisions for staff and postdoctoral researchers on R01 or RPG awards and have the ability to hire non-citizens with appropriate visa status. In 2016, 10 percent of postdoctoral researchers in the biomedical, behavioral, social, and clinical sciences were supported by federal traineeships and fellowships, whereas 46 percent were supported by federal research grants.[48]

In 2003, prior to the release of *Bridges to Independence*, NIH created the Ruth L. Kirschstein Interdisciplinary Research Training Award (T90) combined

---

[45] See https://grants.nih.gov/grants/guide/pa-files/PA-14-044.html (accessed December 11, 2017).
[46] See https://report.nih.gov/NIHDatabook/Charts/Default.aspx?showm=Y&chartId=211&catId=16 (accessed December 11, 2017).
[47] See https://grants.nih.gov/grants/funding/t90.htm (accessed December 11, 2017).
[48] See https://report.nih.gov/NIHDatabook/Charts/Default.aspx?showm=Y&chartId=263&catId=20 (accessed February 28, 2018).

with a Research Education Grant (R90) (discussed in section 1.11), which permits research education experiences for individuals who do not meet the qualification for support under the NRSA program.[49,50]

1.13 NIH should commission an independent evaluation of different models of postdoctoral support.

Bridges to Independence (2005)

Since the release of this recommendation, NIH has conducted various evaluations of postdoctoral support. In 2006, NIH released an independently authored report titled *The Career Achievements of NRSA Postdoctoral Trainees and Fellows* that discussed the value of independent awards for postdoctoral researchers.[51] NIH reported in 2016 that successful RPG awardees are more likely to have previously been supported on an F or T award (either pre-doctoral or postdoctoral).[52] NIH also indicated that the Division of Biomedical Research Workforce (DBRW) is completing an evaluation of the outcomes of F32 fellowship programs between 1996 and 2008.

NIH has been monitoring the progress of its K99 awardees and the extent to which they are identifying appropriate positions, transitioning to the R00 phase of the award, and subsequently applying for R01s. According to NIH, early results have been positive overall. Since its launch, more than 2,000 investigators have received the K99 award.[53] Of the cohort funded in 2007 (183 investigators), 93 percent transitioned into the R00 phase, indicating that they successfully secured an independent research faculty position at an extramural institution within the United States.[54] Of those that transitioned to the R00 stage, 59 percent secured an R01 grant by 2014. These results led to a recommendation from the Advisory Committee to the NIH Director (ACD) working group that studied the biomedical research workforce to increase the number of K99/R00 awards beginning in FY2014.[55]

In 2011, NIH released an independently authored report on an evaluation of outcomes of the NIH Individual Mentored Career Development Award Programs

---

[49] See https://www.law.cornell.edu/cfr/text/42/66.103 (accessed December 11, 2017).

[50] See https://researchtraining.nih.gov/programs/training-grants/T90-R90 (accessed December 11, 2017).

[51] See https://grants.nih.gov/training/nrsa_report_5_16_06-2.doc (accessed February 28, 2018).

[52] See https://nexus.od.nih.gov/all/2016/11/28/how-many-researchers-were-supported-by-nih-as-trainees/ (accessed December 11, 2017).

[53] See https://report.nih.gov/NIHDatabook/Charts/Default.aspx?showm=Y&chartId=211&catId=16 (accessed December 11, 2017).

[54] See http://datahound.scientopia.org/2014/07/17/my-first-pass-evaluation-of-the-k99-r00-program/ (accessed December 11, 2017).

[55] See https://grants.nih.gov/grants/new_investigators/QsandAs.htm#1624 (accessed December 11, 2017).

or K awards.[56] NIH reports that the DBRW is planning a follow-up evaluation of outcomes of these K awards in 2017-2018.

A 2011 study supported by NIH evaluation funds, but conducted by scholars independent of NIH, found positive impacts of NIH postdoctoral training grants on publication statistics.[57] This study found "that for applicants in the neighborhood of the funding cutoff, receipt of an NIH postdoctoral fellowship significantly increases the probability that a new Ph.D. will successfully make the transition to a research career and the number of articles published in the ten years following grant receipt" (p. 12).

2. RECOMMENDATIONS ON SUPPORTING DIVERSITY

Diversity in the biomedical and behavioral research workforce is critical to ensure that the best and brightest minds have the opportunity to contribute to the realization of national research goals. Yet despite longstanding efforts from NIH and other entities across the biomedical and behavioral research landscape to increase the number of scientists from underrepresented groups, diversity in biomedicine still falls short of mirroring that of the U.S. population. These populations include women, people from traditionally underrepresented minority (URM) groups, individuals with disabilities, and people from disadvantaged backgrounds across the lifespan of a research career.

2.1 There is a need for stronger coordination of diversity-related efforts and evaluation of outcomes at NIH.

Biomedical Research Workforce Working Group Report (2012)
Working Group on Diversity in the Biomedical Research Workforce (2012)
Physician-Scientist Workforce Working Group Report (2014)

To address findings in a series of NIH studies on the diversity of the biomedical workforce, including minority underrepresentation in biomedical and behavioral research,[58] NIH director Francis Collins charged the ACD in 2011 to form a Working Group on Diversity in the Biomedical Research Workforce. This working group was asked to examine and develop effective strategies to increase diversity.[59]

In 2013, NIH created a Scientific Workforce Diversity Office under the Office of the Director and recruited a Chief Officer for Scientific Workforce

---

[56] See https://researchtraining.nih.gov/sites/default/files/pdf/K_Awards_Evaluation_FinalReport_20110901.pdf# (accessed December 11, 2017).

[57] See https://www.ncbi.nlm.nih.gov/pmc/articles/PMC3158578/ (accessed December 11, 2017).

[58] See https://www.ncbi.nlm.nih.gov/pubmed/21852498; https://www.ncbi.nlm.nih.gov/pubmed/27306969; https://www.ncbi.nlm.nih.gov/pubmed/23018334; https://papers.ssrn.com/sol3/papers.cfm?abstract_id=1677993 (accessed December 11, 2017).

[59] See https://acd.od.nih.gov/wgd.htm (accessed December 11, 2017).

Diversity (COSWD).[60] That same year, NIH established the Diversity Program Consortium (DPC), consisting of Building Infrastructure Leading to Diversity (BUILD), the National Research Mentoring Network (NRMN), and the Coordination and Evaluation Center (CEC). The CEC evaluates diversity of the BUILD and NRMN programs.[61] In total, NIH invested $31 million into 12 institutions as part of the collaborating NRMN, BUILD, and CEC awards.[62] This investment in diversity programs is ancillary to existing diversity programs operational in the various NIH Institutes and Centers. While the CEC has been established, the results of its work have not been finalized and made public.

In 2016, the Scientific Workforce Diversity Officer in the Office for Extramural Programs and a trans-NIH working group developed and launched a website that consolidates information and opportunities available to individuals from underrepresented backgrounds interested in biomedical careers.[63] The Reports and Data section of the website provides links to data repositories and reports that capture trends in diversity, the scientific workforce, and U.S. Census data.[64]

2.2 NIH should partner with established minority scientific and professional groups to implement a system of mentorship networks for underrepresented minority students.
Working Group on Diversity in the Biomedical Research Workforce (2012)

A nationwide consortium of biomedical professionals and institutions established the NRMN in 2014 to develop a national network for mentors and mentees in biomedical research. NRMN partners with institutions and professional societies/organizations across the nation to diversify the biomedical workforce by (1) Increasing access to mentoring across all career stages; (2) Training mentors, grant writing coaches, and mentees with a focus on cultural responsiveness; (3) Increasing access to research resources and career development opportunities; and (4) Advancing the science of mentoring.

2.3 NIH should establish a working group of the ACD of racially and ethnically diverse scientists to provide regular input to the Director of NIH and Institutes regarding the state-of-the-art in effective programs that reduce disparities in research awards.
Working Group on Diversity in the Biomedical Research Workforce (2012)

---

[60] See https://diversity.nih.gov/ (accessed December 11, 2017).

[61] See https://commonfund.nih.gov/diversity/overview (accessed December 11, 2017).

[62] See https://nrmnet.net/the-nih-diversity-program-consortium-integration-of-nrmn-cec-build/ (accessed December 11, 2017).

[63] See https://extramural-diversity.nih.gov/ (accessed December 11, 2017).

[64] See http://extramural-diversity.nih.gov/diversity-reports (accessed December 11, 2017).

NIH formed a subcommittee of the ACD Working Group on Diversity on peer review, which held a competition in 2014 to generate ideas to detect bias and strengthen fairness and impartiality in peer review.[65] In addition, NIH is currently piloting anonymization of grant applications.[66] A 2016 NIH report found that disparities in funding continue to persist.[67] For example, the odds of an application from an African-American scientist being funded are 30 percent lower than an application from a white scientist.

2.4 NIH should support infrastructure development of under-resourced institutions with underrepresented minority scientists.
Working Group on Diversity in the Biomedical Research Workforce (2012)

The BUILD program (section 2-1) supports institutional and faculty development in under-resourced institutions, including minority-serving institutions. The SCORE program makes research awards to institutions with historical missions or track records focused on training and graduating students from groups nationally underrepresented in biomedical research.[68]

Another NIH program supporting under-resourced institutions is the AREA award (R15), which provides research grants to PIs at institutions that are not major recipients of NIH support. This program has been in place since 1985.[69]

2.5 NIH should appoint a Chief Diversity Officer and establish an Office of Diversity.
Working Group on Diversity in the Biomedical Research Workforce (2012)

NIH established the Scientific Workforce Diversity Office (SWD) in 2013, and Dr. Hannah Valantine became COSWD in March 2014. NIH deliberately specified that the COSWD must be a practicing scientist, and Valantine has an intramural lab in the National Heart, Lung, and Blood Institute (NHLBI), where she pursues clinical research in cardiology.

2.6 NIH should institute a comprehensive search process to diversify intramural tenure-track investigators.
Working Group on Diversity in the Biomedical Research Workforce (2012)

---

[65] See https://acd.od.nih.gov/prsub.htm (accessed December 11, 2017).

[66] See https://nexus.od.nih.gov/all/2014/05/29/new-efforts-to-maximize-fairness-in-nih-peer-review/ (accessed December 11, 2017).

[67] See https://diversity.nih.gov/building-evidence/racial-disparities-nih-funding (accessed December 11, 2017).

[68] See https://www.nigms.nih.gov/Research/CRCB/SCORE/Pages/default.aspx (accessed December 11, 2017).

[69] See https://grants.nih.gov/grants/guide/pa-files/PA-03-053.html (accessed December 11, 2017).

Thus far, there is no known action to institute a comprehensive search as recommended. The SWD team has taken some action on projects aiming to diversify the intramural NIH scientific workforce. These efforts involve an integrated strategy to enhance recruitment and retention of diverse faculty in the NIH intramural research program (IRP). One strategy focuses on developing and using a recruitment tool to increase the diversity of the NIH faculty applicant pool.[70] Starting in 2016, NIH IRP also hosted a conference—the Future Research Leaders Conference (FRLC)—to bring highly qualified diverse talent to the NIH campus during the fall NIH Research Festival.[71] NIH expects this to be an annual conference. Additionally, the NIH SWD group developed implicit-bias education modules for presentations and workshops that explain the concept of implicit bias and present scientific evidence of how such bias may affect judgments and decision-making in scientific contexts.[72]

2.7 RPGs funding graduate student and postdoctoral researcher training should be required to provide information on efforts to increase diversity, as training grants currently do.
Research Training in the Biomedical, Behavioral and Clinical Research Sciences (2011)

The current NIH RPG grant criteria for awards contain no requirement for reporting information on efforts to increase diversity.[73] As mentioned in the recommendation, training grants such as T32s do require a recruitment plan to enhance diversity. Peer reviewers evaluate the plan after the overall score has been determined and require modification of proposals with unacceptable plans.[74]

3. RECOMMENDATIONS ON COLLECTING DATA

Broad trends in the training, funding, and employment of early-career researchers are known, but next order data about the changing nature of research positions, career aspirations, and the prospects for the next generation of investigators are incomplete. Informative and disaggregated data on the biomedical workforce could identify trends in career interests and outcomes of graduate students and postdocs, as well as inform institutional and federal policy. To be usable by all stakeholders, these data would need to be made publicly available and accessible.

---

[70] See https://diversity.nih.gov/programs-partnerships (accessed December 11, 2017).
[71] See https://diversity.nih.gov/programs-partnerships/frlc (accessed December 11, 2017).
[72] See https://diversity.nih.gov/programs-partnerships (accessed December 11, 2017).
[73] See https://grants.nih.gov/grants/peer/critiques/rpg.htm (accessed December 11, 2017).
[74] See https://grants.nih.gov/grants/peer/critiques/t32_D.htm (accessed December 11, 2017).

3.1 Institutions should collect data on outcomes of their graduate students and postdoctoral researchers and make that data publicly available. Such information should include completion rates, time to degree, and career outcomes for Ph.D. trainees, as well as time in training and career outcomes from postdoctoral researchers over a 15-year period.

Bridges to Independence (2005)
Biomedical Research Workforce Working Group Report (2012)
Postdoctoral Experience Revisited (2014)
Sustaining Discovery in Biological and Medical Sciences (2015)

Thus far, there is uneven implementation of this recommendation. Graduate and medical schools track information at varying levels of detail and frequency and make it publicly available to varying degrees. Multiple university administrators who presented to the committees spoke to these different approaches to data collection and release. Some institutions collected and published graduate student and/or postdoctoral data before the release of these reports, and there is no clear evidence that tracking expanded in response to these recommendations. Examples of institutions collecting graduate and postdoctoral data and sharing it with the public include the University of California, Berkeley, Stanford University, University of California, San Francisco, and University of Michigan.[75]

Following the *Bridges to Independence* report, the NIH Health Reform Act of 2006 (P.L.109-482) was signed into law. Section 403C of the law stipulates that institutions receiving NIH-funded training grants are required to report doctoral completion rates and time to degree annually to both the NIH director and applicants to graduate programs at those institutions. In 2009, this requirement was added to the program statistics section of NIH Training Data Tables, which universities must complete to renew training grants, and became a new assurance requirement, which universities must fulfill in order to be eligible for training grants.[76,77,78] However, the recommendations outlined in the latter three reports pointed to the inadequacy of these data in helping students make educational and

---

[75] See https://graduate.ucsf.edu/aggregate-data; http://web.stanford.edu/dept/pres-provost/irds/Ph.D.jobs; http://grad.berkeley.edu/doctoral-alumni-outcomes/placement-survey/; https://secure.rackham.umich.edu/academic_information/program_statistics/ (accessed December 11, 2017).

[76] See https://www.congress.gov/109/plaws/publ482/PLAW-109publ482.pdf (accessed December 11, 2017).

[77] See https://grants.nih.gov/grants/guide/notice-files/NOT-OD-09-141.html (accessed December 11, 2017).

[78] In 2015, NIH released a series of new data tables for institutions receiving NIH training grants to complete in conjunction with their applications and progress reports. These data tables ask that institutions collect and report the following information for their trainees: degree completion and dates, career outcomes, and research support over a 15-year period. See https://grants.nih.gov/grants/guide/notice-files/NOT-OD-15-112.html and https://grants.nih.gov/grants/guide/notice-files/NOT-OD-16-007.html (accessed December 11, 2017).

career decisions. For example, the 2015 *Sustaining Discovery* report cited a need for information on career outcomes for graduate students and for basic information such as postdoctoral researchers' time in training to be made available, but these data are not yet required.

As the *Biomedical Research Workforce Working Group Report* articulated, "aggregate level data [are] necessary to determine the number of people in various positions, but individual-level data and longitudinal individual data would make it possible to identify the characteristics and trajectories of individuals and is important for rigorous modeling and evaluation." As this report points out, NSF's Graduate Student Survey, Survey of Earned Doctorates, and Survey of Doctorate Recipients omit large portions of the postdoctoral population for structural reasons. In addition, these surveys include only doctorate-granting institutions, not research centers and national labs, and only U.S.-trained doctorates. NSF's Scientists and Engineers Statistical Data System (SESTAT) and Bureau of Labor Statistics Occupational Employment Statistics (BLS OES) data also have limitations for gathering data on industrial employment of biomedical researchers, including a 4-year lag and no disaggregation by education level.

The following summarizes specific data recommendations—not responses—by report:

- *Sustaining Discovery in Biological and Medical Sciences*: Institutions should publish data on career outcomes of each department's graduate students and postdocs. This information should be readily available to prospective graduate students and applicants. Institutions can collect this information using their fundraising offices and social media resources. This information should include completion rate, time to degree, career outcomes for Ph.D. trainees, and time in training and career outcomes from postdoctoral researchers over a 15-year period. Each institution should collect and prominently display this information on its website.
- *The Postdoctoral Experience Revisited*: Every institution that employs postdoctoral researchers should collect data on the number of currently employed postdocs and where they go after completion and should make this information publicly available. NSF should serve as the primary curator for establishing and updating a database system that tracks postdoctoral researchers, including non-academic and foreign trained postdocs. Host institutions should be consistent with their labeling of postdoctoral researchers, keep track of new hires and departures, and conduct exit interviews to determine career outcomes, and they should make this information available publicly. This activity should be coordinated through a postdoctoral office and take advantage of new technology, including social media.
- *Biomedical Research Workforce Working Group Report*: Institutions receiving NIH funding should collect information on the career outcomes of both their graduate students and postdoctoral researchers and provide

this information to prospective students and postdoctoral researchers and NIH. Such information should include completion rates, time to degree, career outcomes for Ph.D. trainees, and time in training and career outcomes from postdoctoral researchers over a 15-year period. Institutions should display these outcome data prominently on their websites. This will require institutions to track the career paths of their students and postdoctoral researchers over the long-term. One way to do this would be for an institution to assign graduate students and incoming postdoctoral researchers an identifier, or to use an identifier such as ORCID,[79] that it can then use to track its graduate students and postdocs throughout their careers. This could be part of a unique researcher identification (ID) system that would allow tracking of all researchers throughout their career. The ID would need to relate to any NIH ID assigned to the individual.

- *Bridges to Independence*: Data about all career stages of the biomedical workforce must include the growing population of staff scientists and other non-tenure-track researchers. Moreover, data collection strategies should also be constructed to allow for disaggregated information to detect different trends between sub-populations of the biomedical research workforce. The committee encourages institutions to collect and make available information about the career outcomes of recent postdoctoral researchers.

3.2 NIH, NSF, and other federal agencies should address data gaps and collect ongoing information on the biomedical and scientific workforce.

Bridges to Independence (2005)
Biomedical Research Workforce Working Group Report (2012)
Working Group on Diversity in the Biomedical Research Workforce report (2012)
Physician-Scientist Workforce Working Group Report (2014)
The Postdoctoral Experience Revisited (2014)

Using the eRA Commons ID and Research Performance Progress Report (RPPR), NIH started tracking postdoctoral researchers participating in NIH-funded grants in 2009 and graduate students participating in NIH-funded grants in 2013.[80,81] NIH has also automated the tabulation of the subsequent institutions and grants of trainees on training grants, degree completion and dates, career out-

---

[79] See https://orcid.org/ (accessed December 11, 2017).
[80] See https://grants.nih.gov/grants/guide/notice-files/NOT-OD-09-140.html (accessed December 11, 2017).
[81] See https://grants.nih.gov/grants/guide/notice-files/NOT-OD-13-097.html (accessed December 11, 2017).

comes, and research support over a 15-year period.[82] NIH developed the SciENcv network to help researchers update their CVs as well as keep track of researchers' activities.[83] NIH also supported the development of IPUMS Higher Ed, a publicly available tool released in 2016 that harmonizes multiple NSF datasets—the National and International Survey of Doctoral Recipients (SDR) databases and Survey of College Graduates (NSCG) and National Survey of Recent College Graduates (NSRCG) databases—from 1990 to 2013. This system provides a user-friendly data extraction system to track career trajectories of Ph.D.'s across different occupations, including in academia, government, industry, and other types of research involvement.

NSF and NIH co-sponsored the development of a Survey of Postdocs at Federally Funded Research Development Centers in 2005 and piloted a Survey of Early Career Doctorates in 2015 to understand the employment of individuals who earned doctorates within the past 10 years.[84,85] A summary of the Survey of Early Career Doctorates is available, and detailed data are forthcoming.[86] While these data collection tools take major steps in the recommended direction, additional efforts may be required to fully address and define workforce data needs.

3.3 NIH should create a permanent unit in the Office of the Director that works with the extramural research community to coordinate data collection and analysis of the workforce and evaluate NIH policies.
Biomedical Research Workforce Working Group Report (2012)

NIH established DBRW in 2013 to collect and analyze biomedical research workforce data. DBRW works with the Office of Director through the Office of Extramural Research.[87]

4. RECOMMENDATIONS TO SUPPORT EARLY-CAREER INVESTIGATORS

The success of the biomedical research enterprise depends on the uninterrupted entry of well-trained, skilled, and motivated scientists. However, recent trends in employment and funding opportunities reflect a hypercompetitive atmo-

---

[82] See https://era.nih.gov/services_for_applicants/other/xTract.cfm; https://grants.nih.gov/grants/guide/notice-files/NOT-OD-15-112.html; https://grants.nih.gov/grants/guide/notice-files/NOT-OD-16-007.html (accessed December 11, 2017).
[83] See https://www.ncbi.nlm.nih.gov/sciencv/ (accessed December 11, 2017).
[84] See https://www.nsf.gov/statistics/srvyffrdcpd/#sd (accessed December 11, 2017).
[85] See https://www.nsf.gov/statistics/srvyecd/#sd&tabs-1 (accessed December 11, 2017).
[86] See https://www.nsf.gov/statistics/srvyecd/ (accessed December 11, 2017).
[87] See https://biomedicalresearchworkforce.nih.gov/create-office.htm (accessed December 11, 2017).

sphere for independent research careers, potentially dissuading or discouraging trained researchers from remaining in biomedical research after years of training.

4.1 NIH should address the gap in RPG award rates between new and established investigators.
Physician-Scientist Workforce Working Group Report (2014)

The success rates of new and established investigators receiving R01 funding equivalent to an RPG, where "new" denotes investigators who have not previously received an R award, was 14 percent vs. 16 percent, respectively, in 2014; 16 percent in both groups in 2015; and 16 percent vs. 18 percent in 2016. It is unclear whether there is a consistent gap in success rates to address (Figure B-8), though the absolute number of established investigators supported on R01s is markedly greater than that of new investigators (Figure B-9).

NIH is aware of concerns that the percentage of mid-career investigators with RPGs has been declining in recent years[88] and has recently proposed limitations to the research funding provided to individual investigators to partially address this.[89] NIH also recently proposed a Next Generation Researcher Initiative, which addresses concerns about mid-career investigators.[90]

4.2 NIH should double the number of NIH Director's Early Independence awards.
Biomedical Research Workforce Working Group Report (2012)

The number of Director's Early Independence (DP5) awards, which fund doctoral-level researchers directly entering independent research careers without a postdoctoral training period, grew from 10 in 2011 to 16 in 2016, which is an increase but not a doubling.[91]

4.3 NIH should establish a program to promote innovative research by scientists transitioning into their first independent positions. These grants would replace the K22 awards, and NIH should make 200 grants annually of $500,000 each, payable over 5 years.
Bridges to Independence (2005)

---

[88] See http://journals.plos.org/plosone/article?id=10.1371/journal.pone.0168511 (accessed December 11, 2017).

[89] See https://www.nih.gov/about-nih/who-we-are/nih-director/statements/new-nih-approach-grant-funding-aimed-optimizing-stewardship-taxpayer-dollars (accessed December 11, 2017).

[90] See https://www.nih.gov/about-nih/who-we-are/nih-director/statements/launching-next-generation-researchers-initiative-strengthen-biomedical-research-enterprise (accessed December 11, 2017).

[91] See https://report.nih.gov/success_rates/Success_ByActivity.cfm (accessed December 11, 2017).

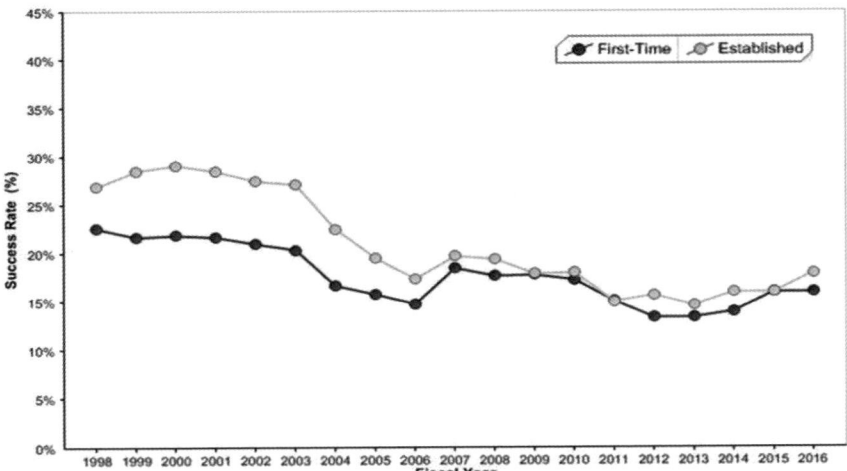

FIGURE B-8 Success rates for new (type1) R01-equivalent grants, by career stage of investigator.
SOURCE: NIH Data Book.

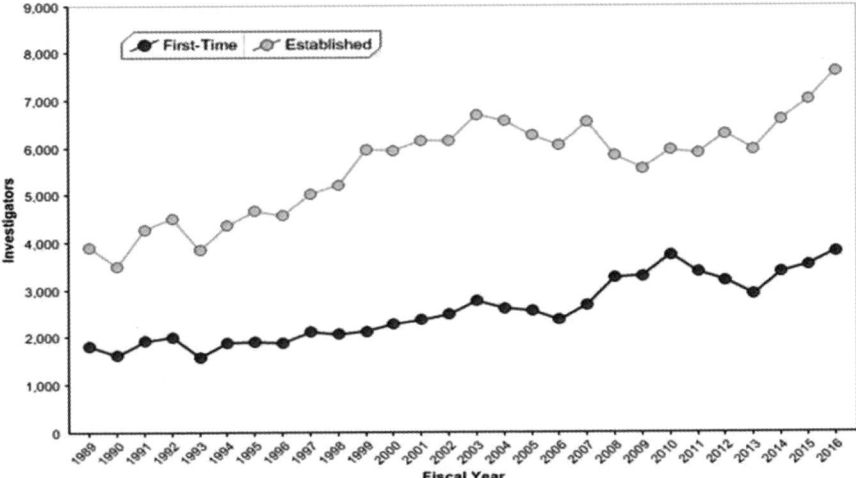

FIGURE B-9 Number of investigators supported on competing research project grants, by career stage of investigator.
SOURCE: NIH Data Book.

There is no indication that the K22 award program has been fully removed or replaced among NIH Institutes, and many Institutes still support the K22.[92] However, NIH initiated the Pathway to Independence awards (K99 and R00) in 2007 in response to this recommendation and awards approximately 200 K99s each year in accordance with the recommendation. In the K99 phase of the award, the awardee receives salary up to $100,000 per year, plus fringe benefits, and research support up to $25,000 per year that may vary by the awarding institute.[93] In the R00 phase of the award, the awardee receives total costs of $249,000 per year for up to 3 years, half of the recommended funding level.[94]

4.4 NIH should establish a New Investigator R01 grant where the "preliminary results" section is replaced by "previous experience" to encourage higher-risk proposals.

Bridges to Independence (2005)

The NIH Director's New Innovator Award (DP2) has existed specifically for early-career researchers since 2007, and in August 2012 NIH clarified in the funding opportunity description that the emphasis for this award is on innovation rather than preliminary data. The total funding dedicated to these awards is $80 million for 33 awards in FY2017,[95] a funding level that has changed over time—for example, $106 million funded 45 awards in 2015, and $132 million funded 56 awards in 2016.[96]

As of 2009, NIH reviews R01 equivalent grant applications from new or early-stage investigators separately from grant applications from established investigators. NIH advises reviewers to expect less preliminary data from new investigators than they do from more experienced PIs.[97,98]

---

[92] See http://grants.nih.gov/grants/guide/rfa-files/RFA-DC-15-002; http://grants.nih.gov/grants/guide/pa-files/PAR-16-140.html; http://grants.nih.gov/grants/guide/pa-files/PAR-16-220.html; http://grants.nih.gov/grants/guide/pa-files/PAR-16-267.html; http://grants.nih.gov/grants/guide/pa-files/PAR-16-293.html; http://grants.nih.gov/grants/guide/pa-files/PAR-16-340.html; http://grants.nih.gov/grants/guide/pa-files/PAR-16-389.html; http://grants.nih.gov/grants/guide/pa-files/PAR-16-434.html; http://grants.nih.gov/grants/guide/pa-files/PAR-17-069.html (accessed December 11, 2017).

[93] See https://grants.nih.gov/grants/guide/contacts/parent_K99_R00.html (accessed December 11, 2017).

[94] See https://www.nhlbi.nih.gov/research/training/programs/postdoc/pathway-parent-k99-r00 (accessed December 11, 2017).

[95] See https://grants.nih.gov/grants/guide/rfa-files/RFA-RM-16-004.html (accessed December 11, 2017).

[96] See https://report.nih.gov/success_rates/Success_ByActivity.cfm (accessed December 11, 2017).

[97] See https://grants.nih.gov/policy/new_investigators/index.htm (accessed December 11, 2017).

[98] See https://grants.nih.gov/grants/guide/notice-files/NOT-OD-09-013.html (accessed December 11, 2017).

4.5 NIH should establish a physician-scientist-specific granting mechanism to facilitate transitions to research independence. This program should be similar to the K99/R00 program.
   Physician-Scientist Workforce Working Group Report (2014)

NIH released a Request for Information in 2014 to assess how a K99/R00 program for physician-scientists would work.[99] In 2016 NIH added a section to the K99/R00 Funding Opportunity Announcement stating explicitly that physician-scientists are eligible to apply.[100] In August 2017 NIH announced that National Institute of Allergy and Infectious Diseases (NIAID) is offering a physician-scientist-targeted version of the K99/R00.[101]

K08 and K23 awards are individual career development awards for physician-scientists and are designed to provide a period of mentored research and a pathway to research independence.[102] They differ from the K99-R00 in that they do not have a linked individual R00 award.

In 2016, NIH hosted three workshops to discuss potential new initiatives to support physician-scientists. The discussions at these workshops contributed to a paper in *Academic Medicine* describing recommended initiatives (in press).

4.6 NIH should double the number of Pathway to Independence awards (K99/R00) and shorten eligibility for applying from five years to three years of postdoctoral experience.
   Biomedical Research Workforce Working Group Report (2012)

As of 2014, eligible K99 applicants must have fewer than 4 years of postdoctoral experience, down from fewer than 5 years in 2011. This change was intended to hasten the transition to independence.[103] The number of K99 awards has increased, but not doubled, since the release of the report in 2012 (Figure B-1).[104]

4.7 NIH should expand the K24 mentoring award mechanism to include basic sciences and adapt the award to provide opportunities for mid-career faculty to mentor early-stage investigators.
   Research Training in the Biomedical, Behavioral and Clinical Research Sciences (2011)

---

[99] See https://grants.nih.gov/grants/guide/notice-files/NOT-OD-15-009.html (accessed December 11, 2017).
[100] See https://grants.nih.gov/grants/guide/pa-files/PA-16-077.html (accessed December 11, 2017).
[101] See https://grants.nih.gov/grants/guide/pa-files/PAR-17-329.html (accessed December 11, 2017).
[102] See https://grants.nih.gov/grants/guide/notice-files/NOT-OD-15-009.html# (accessed December 11, 2017).
[103] See http://www.sciencemag.org/careers/2013/05/nihs-pathway-independence-award-aims-younger (accessed December 11, 2017).
[104] See http://www.sciencemag.org/careers/2013/05/nihs-pathway-independence-award-aims-younger (accessed December 11, 2017).

Not all NIH Institutes offer the patient-oriented K24 award. For example, the National Institute of Diabetes and Digestive and Kidney Diseases (NIDDK) withdrew from participation in 2017, and the National Eye Institute (NEI), National Institute of Biomedical Imaging and Bioengineering (NIBIB), and National Institute of Dental and Craniofacial Research (NIDCR) have not participated since 2009.[105,106]

Currently, there is no mid-career investigator mentoring award for basic research, and no apparent move or Request for Information to begin the process.

4.8 NIH should establish a renewable R01-like grant for small science projects (<$100k) open to researchers who do not have PI status on another research grant.

Bridges to Independence (2005)

Currently, NIH does not provide a renewable R01-like grant for small research projects.

NIH's R03 grant was established in 2003, prior to the report release. It supports small pilot projects of under $50,000 and less than 2 years, but it does not specify the PI's grant status, is not renewable, and is smaller than this report recommends. The *Bridges to Independence* report noted that R03s are "generally not sufficient for supporting an entire research laboratory, leading new investigators attracted to such programs—because of the lack of preliminary data—scrambling to find funding from many different sources."

4.9 Non tenure track "soft money" researchers should have a budgetary safety net that provides time to reapply for grant support if their funding lapses. The NIH contribution to this safety net should be expanding R55 Shannon awards to provide merit-based bridge awards.

Bridges to Independence (2005)

In 2005, the R56 High Priority Short Term Award replaced the R55 Shannon Award, which had provided $100,000 over 2 years to PIs whose grant applications were scored highly but not funded, to strengthen their proposals for resubmission. The R56 award also provides interim funding of up to 2 years and includes support for gathering data to reapply for NIH research grants. In 2004, the year before report release, NIH funded 10 R56 awards at a total award amount

---

[105] See https://grants.nih.gov/grants/guide/pa-files/PA-09-037.html; https://grants.nih.gov/grants/guide/pa-files/PA-10-061.html; https://grants.nih.gov/grants/guide/pa-files/PA-14-047.html; https://grants.nih.gov/grants/guide/pa-files/PA-16-206.html; https://grants.nih.gov/grants/guide/notice-files/NOT-DK-17-005.html (accessed December 11, 2017).

[106] A list of current participating Institutes is available at https://grants.nih.gov/grants/guide/pa-files/PA-16-206.html (accessed December 11, 2017).

of $500,000. In FY2016, NIH funded a total of 332 R56 grants at a total award amount of $146,697,228, representing a significant expansion of the bridge award mechanism.[107,108]

4.10 NIH should expand loan repayment programs to all students pursuing biomedical physician-scientist researcher careers and increase the amount of loans forgiven to reflect the debt burden of current trainees.

Physician-Scientist Workforce Working Group Report (2014)

In 2015, 1 year after the report release, the NIH Loan Repayment Program (LRP) contributed $360,000 in additional funds toward these 2-year awards for physician-scientists, funding approximately the same number of applicants at the same mean award level of $51,000. For comparison, 79 percent of new award recipients had educational debt greater than $50,000. However, 2015 is the last year NIH released LRP data, and it is possible that funding levels have changed since then.[109]

In 2016, the 21st Century Cures Act (P.L. 114-255) authorized increases in the amount of LRP to a maximum of $50,000 per year and granted the NIH director authority to expand the number of LRPs to reflect workforce and research needs.[110] NIH does not appear to have expanded access by physician-scientists to LRPs beyond the current programs for which they are eligible: clinical research, pediatric research, health disparities research, contraception and infertility research, and clinical research for individuals from disadvantaged backgrounds.[111]

5. RECOMMENDATIONS TO SUPPORT FACULTY

As research funding becomes increasingly hypercompetitive, even highly productive faculty researchers with established records of success with NIH grants may experience lengthy gaps in renewal support, thereby disrupting successful research careers and sometimes even leading to closure of research laboratories. Lower success rates lead faculty researchers to devote more of their time to writing proposals, which in turn leads to more time and effort expended in the grant procurement process instead of research.

5.1 NIH should consider a long-term approach to reduce the percentage of funds from NIH sources used for faculty salary support.

Biomedical Research Workforce Working Group Report (2012)

---

[107] See https://grants.nih.gov/grants/funding/r56.htm (accessed December 11, 2017).
[108] See https://report.nih.gov/success_rates/Success_ByActivity.cfm (accessed December 11, 2017).
[109] See https://www.lrp.nih.gov/data-reports (accessed December 11, 2017).
[110] See https://www.congress.gov/114/bills/hr6/BILLS-114hr6rfs.pdf (accessed December 11, 2017).
[111] See https://www.lrp.nih.gov/data-reports (accessed December 11, 2017).

In July 2013, NIH administered a pilot survey at nine institutions to obtain data on the percentage of salary covered by NIH grant dollars, but NIH has not taken any policy actions since the survey. NIH indicated to the committee its concerns about the burden on respondents completing the survey and the variability in levels of soft-money support across different types of faculty positions and different types of institutions, such as research hospitals, institutions without a medical school, and independent research institutes. NIH does not anticipate collecting additional data.[112] This type of data is being collected directly through U-Metrics, and expansion of those efforts will eventually provide detailed information about the proportion of salary derived from federal grants.

The National Institute of General Medical Sciences' (NIGMS) Maximizing Investigator Research Awards (MIRA; R35) program recommends that, "Because most institutions expect some commitment from investigators to administrative, teaching and/or clinical duties, any salary support for the Program Director (PD)/PI requested on the grant should generally be less than 51 percent of the PD/PI's annual salary and should in no case be more than the actual research effort the PD/PI will devote to the grant."[113] Individual NIH Institutes have different policies on this; the R35 administered by the National Cancer Institute (NCI),[114] for example, suggests but does not require that institutions will commit 20 percent of PI salary, and the R35 administered by the National Institute of Neurological Disorders and Stroke (NINDS)[115] has no stipulation on salary support.

5.2 Congress should increase the NIH salary cap contingent upon a reduced Facilities and Administrative (F&A) cost recovery at higher salary levels.

Sustaining Discovery in Biological and Medical Sciences (2015)

The NIH salary cap is set by appropriations law at Executive Level II of the Federal Executive pay scale. The NIH Executive Level II salary cap was increased from $183,300 to $185,100 under the Consolidated Appropriations Act, effective January 10, 2016, and to $187,000 effective January 8, 2017. However, this is in line with previous annual increases, and it does not take into account a reduced F&A cost recovery.[116] Congress has not passed legislation related to reduced F&A cost recovery at higher salary levels.[117]

---

[112] See https://biomedicalresearchworkforce.nih.gov/discussion.htm (accessed December 11, 2017).

[113] See https://grants.nih.gov/grants/guide/pa-files/PAR-17-094.html; https://grants.nih.gov/grants/guide/pa-files/PAR-17-190.html (accessed December 11, 2017).

[114] See https://grants.nih.gov/grants/guide/pa-files/PAR-16-411.html (accessed December 11, 2017).

[115] See https://grants.nih.gov/grants/guide/rfa-files/RFA-NS-17-020.html (accessed December 11, 2017).

[116] See https://grants.nih.gov/grants/guide/notice-files/NOT-OD-16-045.html; https://grants.nih.gov/grants/guide/notice-files/NOT-OD-17-048.html (accessed December 11, 2017).

[117] See https://grants.nih.gov/grants/guide/notice-files/NOT-OD-16-045.html (accessed December 11, 2017).

6. RECOMMENDATIONS TO SUPPORT STAFF SCIENTISTS

The U.S. biomedical workforce depends heavily on the labor of temporary trainees, such as graduate students and postdocs, leading to the current disequilibrium in the research enterprise given that few academic research positions exist for these trained researchers to enter. To address this imbalance and promote sustainability in the workforce, some groups have suggested the greater utilization of staff scientists in lieu of trainees. Staff scientist positions are non-training positions for Ph.D. scientists interested in running a core facility or serving as a senior researcher in one or multiple laboratories.

6.1 Encourage NIH study sections to be receptive to grant applications that include staff scientists and urge institutions to create position categories that reflect the value and stature of these researchers.
Biomedical Research Workforce Working Group Report (2012)

NIH implemented a change in the instructions to reviewers that directs them to focus on qualifications of applicants rather than job title.[118]

6.2 The research community should employ more staff scientists and consider more extensive use of career technicians.
Sustaining Discovery in Biological and Medical Sciences (2015)

The committee was unable to find evidence of a systematic change in the employment of staff scientists and career technicians in the research community stemming from this recommendation. On November 4, 2016, NIH announced a pilot program to fund the salary and some travel expenses of 50 to 60 staff scientists over 18 months using the R50 "research specialist" award.[119]

In 2015, NIH examined research grant progress reports and determined that NIH research grants do support a substantial number of staff scientists. NIH examined the 50,885 grant projects funded in FY2009 and identified 23,329 individuals, out of the 247,457 total individuals on grants, with the title staff scientist.[120]

7. RECOMMENDATIONS ON GRANT REVIEW

Since 1946, the expert review by scientific peers has guided NIH funding of scientists in biomedical research. In 2009, NIH introduced a set of five

---

[118] See https://biomedicalresearchworkforce.nih.gov/encourage.htm (accessed December 11, 2017).
[119] See http://www.sciencemag.org/news/2015/03/cancer-institute-plans-new-award-staff-scientists; https://grants.nih.gov/grants/guide/pa-files/PAR-17-049.html (accessed December 11, 2017).
[120] See http://www.fasebj.org/content/early/2015/11/30/fj.14-264358.full.pdf (accessed December 11, 2017).

criteria—approach, significance, investigator, innovation, and environment—to guide the peer review of grant applications. The most meritorious applications are discussed by a study section of reviewers composed of research peers who then assign scores for each of the criteria and an overall impact score. There is no absolute correspondence between the impact score of a proposal and whether NIH funds it. In its report, the Working Group on Diversity in the Biomedical Research Workforce acknowledged that peer review is an imprecise tool for selecting awards, and in light of the existence of some evidence suggesting that peer review may be subject to reviewer biases, called for further exploration of peer review and its impact on the workforce.

7.1 NIH should establish a new Working Group of the ACD composed of experts in behavioral and social sciences and studies of diversity with a special focus on determining and combating real or perceived biases in the NIH peer review system.
Working Group on Diversity in the Biomedical Research Workforce (2012)

NIH established the ACD Diversity Working Group Subcommittee on Peer Review in response to this recommendation. The Subcommittee on Peer Review is charged with examining all hypotheses, including the role of unconscious bias, related to disparities in research awards at NIH (see section 2-3). The subcommittee will provide advice on potential interventions to ensure the fairness of the peer review system.[121]

7.2 NIH should design an experiment to determine the effects of anonymizing applications with respect to applicant identity as well as that of an applicant's institution.
Working Group on Diversity in the Biomedical Research Workforce (2012)

NIH indicated in 2012, after this recommendation was made, that it intended to pilot a program to anonymize applications[122] and indicated in 2014 that these tests were in progress.[123] NIH has not released the results. In addition, the Center for Scientific Review (CSR) created two challenges to elicit proposals on New Methods to Detect Bias in Peer Review and Strategies to Strengthen Fairness and Impartiality in Peer Review. CSR chose winners in September 2014 but has not yet posted the results of these challenges.[124]

---

[121] See https://acd.od.nih.gov/prsub.htm (accessed December 11, 2017).

[122] See https://www.nih.gov/news-events/nih-proposes-critical-initiatives-sustain-future-us-biomedical-research (accessed December 11, 2017).

[123] See https://nexus.od.nih.gov/all/2014/05/29/new-efforts-to-maximize-fairness-in-nih-peer-review/ (accessed December 11, 2017).

[124] See https://nexus.od.nih.gov/all/2014/05/29/new-efforts-to-maximize-fairness-in-nih-peer-review/ (accessed December 11, 2017).

7.3 NIH should pilot different forms of validated implicit bias/ diversity awareness training for NIH scientific review officers and program officers to determine the most efficacious approaches.
Working Group on Diversity in the Biomedical Research Workforce (2012)

The NIH SWD group developed implicit bias education modules for presentations and workshops (see section 2-6). The COSWD has indicated that approximately 300 investigators have received this training as of 2017,[125] though it is unclear what roles those investigators held in the grant review process. In addition, CSR created two challenges to maximize fairness in peer review of grant applications (see section 7-2).

---

[125] See https://diversity.nih.gov/blog/2017-04-19-re-thinking-first-impressions (accessed December 11, 2017).

C

Dear Colleague Letter

The National Academies of
SCIENCES · ENGINEERING · MEDICINE

Thursday, August 03, 2017

Dear Colleague,

The Next Generation Researchers Initiative Committee of the National Academies of Sciences, Engineering, and Medicine invites your input on effective, systemic strategies to ensure the successful launch and sustainment of research careers in the biomedical and behavioral sciences.

This initiative was requested by the U.S. Congress in the 2016 Appropriations Act (Public Law 114-113) that directed the National Institutes of Health (NIH) to contract with the National Academies to produce "(A) an evaluation of the legislative, administrative, educational, and cultural barriers faced by the next generation of researchers; (B) an evaluation of the impact of Federal budget constraints on the next generation of researchers; and (C) recommendations for the implementation of policies to incentivize, improve entry into, and sustain careers in research for the next generation of researchers, including proposed policies for agencies and academic institutions."

The committee is examining evidence-based programs and policies that create more opportunities, incentives, and pathways for successful transitions to independent research careers, as well as factors that influence the stability and sustainability of the early stages of independent research careers.

Request for Information

As a committee of the National Academies, our purpose is to examine the policy and programmatic steps that the nation can undertake to ensure the successful launch and sustainment of careers among the next generation of researchers in the biomedical and behavioral sciences, including the full range of health sciences supported by NIH. We can recommend policy proposals for Congress, federal agencies, academic institutions, state and local government, scientific societies, foundations, and others. We are interested in understanding evaluated or evidence-based practices to improve and incentivize transitions into research independence, particularly actions of university and other non-NIH stakeholders in the enterprise.

As the committee explores the evidence base and potential reforms for the final report, we are seeking input from the full range of stakeholders on the barriers that the next generation of researchers will face as they aspire to and maintain independent research careers in the biomedical and behavioral sciences. We are especially interested in the community's perspective on recommendations offered in previous reports or literature that have not been implemented, and we have highlighted some examples in the subsequent pages. A summary of the larger scope of recommendations from previous reports over the past 20 years examining barriers to the next generation of researchers, "Responses to Prior Report Recommendations," is publicly available to view on the project website, www.nas.edu/NextGen.

In the sections that follow this letter, the committee sketches four broad groups of issues on which we are seeking input. For each group, we provide a brief description of the committee's preliminary understanding of the issues, based on the information we have gathered to date, as well as examples of recommendations that have been suggested by others. This information is not complete but serves as a starting point for comments from the community. We also welcome public input on additional issues or topics that may not be reflected below.

Please send your responses to us by October 1, 2017, via this link: http://www.nas.edu/NextGenInput.

Submitting Input

We look forward to any and all input as we prepare to develop a final report that offers recommendations and promising practices to maintain a high quality, responsive, and vital research enterprise by supporting the next generation of promising biomedical and behavioral researchers.

The information you share will help us gather sufficiently broad input to ensure that we consider all important perspectives and information pertinent to this topic in our deliberations. In addition to requesting your input, we ask you to forward this request for content to those colleagues and thought leaders, as well as affiliated partners in biomedical and behavioral research, who you think might make a unique contribution to this study. Please note that any information you or your colleagues share with the committee will be made public, but anonymous, through our project website, consistent with the Federal Advisory Committee Act.

To allow ample time for the committee to consider your contribution before the drafting and publication of the report, please contribute your input by **October 1, 2017**. If we have follow-up questions regarding your letter, we may contact you by phone or e-mail (if you choose to provide this information). For further information on the study, you may email the study director, Lida Beninson at lbeninson@nas.edu.

Your efforts and input will be greatly appreciated.

On Behalf of the committee,

Ron Daniels

Core Issues for Consideration

I. Level, Sources, and Stability of Research Funding

The U.S. system of biomedical research involves a complex and intricate set of partnerships among the federal government, research universities, scientific societies, foundations and charities, and corporations. However, the portion attributable to the federal government—by far the largest contributor—has declined steadily over time,[1] and NIH funding has fallen more than 15 percent in real dollars from FY 2003 to FY 2017.[2] Most recently, the Administration's 2018 budget proposal includes an additional cut to NIH of more than 20 percent, including roughly a two-thirds reduction in the indirect costs that go to sponsoring institutions.[3]

Although considerable concern has been expressed surrounding the impact of funding reductions on the vigor of the U.S. biomedical research enterprise, we are particularly interested in the impact these reductions would have on the next generation of researchers. For example, some analysts have observed that, because of multi-year commitments, fluctuations in federal funding have had a dramatic effect on the capacity of NIH to award new grants.[4] We have also heard concerns about the effect that the current funding environment may have on the character of the science that is being supported—that it may pose challenges for creative risk-taking, team-based research, and fundamental science.

Examples of recommendations that we have heard from stakeholders, or that have been proposed in the literature, and on which the committee would be interested in the views of the community, include:

- Congress should move to advanced or multi-year appropriations or provide more flexible carry-over authority for the NIH budget.[5]
- Congress should increase the amount of NIH funding that goes to the NIH Common Fund.[6]
- The NIH should expand the number of awards provided through the Director's New Innovator Award Program (DP2).[7]

---

[1] Moses, H. III, et al. (2015). The anatomy of medical research: U.S. and international comparisons, *JAMA 313(2)*, 174-189.

[2] The fiscal year 2017 amount is a preliminary estimate.

[3] Federation of American Sciences for Experimental Biology (FASEB), NIH Appropriations in Current and Constant Dollars, available at http://faseb.org/Portals/2/PDFs/opa/2017/2017Factsheet_Restore%20NIH%20Funding.pdf; Jocelyn Kaiser, NIH plan to reduce overhead payments draws fire, *Science*, June 2, 2017.

[4] Berg, J. Modeling success rates from appropriations histories, *Science*: Sciencehound. August 25, 2016, available at http://blogs.sciencemag.org/sciencehound/2016/08/25/modeling-success-rates/.

[5] Kennedy, J. V., and Atkinson, R.D. (2015). *Healthy Funding: Ensuring a Predictable and Growing Budget for the National Institutes of Health*.

[6] A Vision and Pathway for NIH: Recommendations for the New Administration, November 2016.

[7] Hyman, T., et al. On research funding and the power of youth. ASCB newsletter, October 3, 2016.

- Colleges and universities should revise their criteria for promotion to reduce the emphasis on individual research grant and publication credentials.[8]

II. The Scope of Grant Award and Review

Another focus of our work is the capacity of the U.S. biomedical research enterprise to renew itself. Observers have pointed to a range of evidence to support a concern that the enterprise may be eroding support for the next generation of investigators. For example, the average age to first R01 has increased from 38 years in 1986 to 42 years in 2016.[9] Early career investigators are the principal investigators (PIs) or co-PIs on fewer and smaller grants than other investigators, and so may be more vulnerable to the loss of a grant award on renewal.[10] Further evidence suggests that the aging workforce appears to be drawing grants away from younger investigators, and models demonstrate that the aging of the NIH funded biomedical workforce is likely to continue.[11]

The NIH has intervened over the years to address these trends and the long-term stability of the workforce, including through the introduction of the NIH Pathway to Independence Award (K99/R00), the Director's New Innovator Award Program (DP2), the Directors Early Independence Awards (DP5), and new and ESI programs.[12] Recently, NIH introduced a new Next Generation Researchers Initiative program to reinforce its efforts to bring balance to the workforce.

Separately, the peer review process has come under scrutiny for its possible role in these larger trends. Some studies have suggested that the peer review process may disadvantage underrepresented populations or unconventional ideas.[13] NIH is currently funding studies to further investigate the presence of bias in the peer review process and identify strategies to respond.

Examples of recommendations in these areas that we have heard from stakeholders, or that have been proposed in the literature, and on which the Committee would be interested in the views of the community, are:

---

[8] Casadevall, A., and Fang, F. C. (2012). Reforming science: methodological and cultural reforms. *Infection and Immunity*, *80(3)*, 891-896.

[9] Data provided courtesy of NIH.

[10] Data provided courtesy of NIH.

[11] Blau, D. M., and Weinberg, B. A. (2017). Why the US science and engineering workforce is aging rapidly. *PNAS, 114(15)*, 3879-3884.

[12] More information is available in "Responses to Recommendations in Previous Reports on Biomedical and Behavioral Researchers" at www.nas.edu/NextGen.

[13] National Institutes of Health. 2012. Working Group on Diversity in the Biomedical Research Workforce.

- NIH should modulate the duration of its research project grants to move to either longer[14] or shorter[15] awards, perhaps across the board, or for early-career investigators in particular.
- NIH should alter the K99/R00 program to focus it more specifically on creating opportunities for independent and innovative research.[16]
- NIH should act to limit the number of grant applications per investigator and the turnaround time between submission and decision.[17]

Further, we are interested in the views of the community as to the nature of the programs you would recommend NIH implement through the NGRI program.[18]

III. Training, Mentoring, and Transparency

The trajectory of the next generation of researchers will be defined in no small measure by the trainee experience. The concerns expressed in the community about this aspect of the biomedical enterprise are numerous, including preparation of trainees for non-academic career pathways, and the possible tension between training experiences and labor roles.[19] Regarding postdoctoral positions in particular, previous studies and reports have examined the impacts of salary levels and benefits; prolonged and uncertain postdoctoral periods; inconsistent training opportunities; the absence of formalized career paths for advancement; as well as new evidence suggesting that outside of tenure-track academic jobs, employers do not financially value postdoctoral training.[20]

There are a number of theories in the literature as to the leading causes of these problems. Some say that postdoctoral researchers are not provided adequate data to empower them to make fully informed decisions about their training and career.[21] Others locate the problem in a failure to create pipelines that guide students towards a diversity of biomedical careers.[22] And still others point to deeper, structural problems in the system—for instance, the advocacy group Rescuing Biomedical Research are among those who claim that at the heart of the trainee

---

[14] FASEB. 2015 Sustaining Discovery in Biological and Medical Sciences, A Framework for Discussion.

[15] National Academies Press. (2005). *Bridges to Independence: Fostering the Independence of New Investigators in Biomedical Research.*

[16] Hyman, A. A. (2014). Encouraging innovation. *Molecular Biology of the Cell, 25(4),* 427-428.

[17] Kimble, J., et al. (2015). Strategies from UW-Madison for rescuing biomedical research in the US. *eLIFE 4,* e09305.

[18] NIH Next Generation Researchers Initiative, available at https://grants.nih.gov/ngri.htm.

[19] National Academy of Sciences, National Academy of Engineering, and Institute of Medicine. 2014. *The Postdoctoral Experience Revisited.*

[20] Kahn, S., and Ginther, D. K. (2017). The impact of postdoctoral training on early careers in biomedicine. *Nature Biotechnology, 35(1),* 90-94.

[21] Ibid.

[22] Pickett, C., et al. (2015). Toward a sustainable biomedical research enterprise: Finding consensus and implementing recommendations. *PNAS, 112(35),* 10832-10836.

problem is a misalignment between the number of trainees and the number of available permanent research positions in all sectors.[23]

Examples of recommendations that we have heard from stakeholders, or that have been proposed in the literature, and on which the committee would be interested in the views of the community, are:

- Universities should take action to make available to trainees comprehensive data in areas such as time to degree completion or end of fellowship, salary and benefits, and career outcomes.[24]
- Universities and NIH should actively implement policies to shift from a reliance on postdoctoral fellows and graduate students to staff scientists in research laboratories, including through an expansion of grant programs for staff scientist support.[25]
- NIH should shift to a regime where a far greater number of postdoctoral fellows are supported by training grants or fellowships rather than research grants.[26]

IV. Underrepresented Populations

One area of investigation relates to the challenges certain populations face in entering and developing successful careers in the biomedical research enterprise. The capacity of the system to support the best science will be subverted if systemic barriers thwart the recruitment of the best and brightest scientists irrespective of their race, gender, socioeconomic, or ethnic background. Although the federal government has pursued a range of interventions over the years, and is now actively pursuing additional initiatives in the wake of a 2012 NIH working group report from the Advisory Committee to the Director, studies indicate that we are continuing to fall short of the full objective of achieving diversity in the workforce.[27]

Another vulnerable group in the current biomedical research system is the physician-scientist population. Faced with mounting clinical demands, long training periods, their own unique funding challenges, and an aging workforce, the physician-scientist workforce has declined from 5 percent of all physicians in

---

[23] Alberts, B., et al. (2014). Rescuing US biomedical research from its systemic flaws. *PNAS, 111(16)*, 5773-5777.

[24] Kahn, S., and Ginther, D. K. (2017).

[25] Gibbs, K. D. Jr., et al. (2013). What do I want to be with my Ph.D.? The roles of personal values and structural dynamics in shaping the career interests of recent biomedical science Ph.D. graduates. *CBE- Life Sciences Education 12(4)*, 711-723.

[26] National Institutes of Health (2012). *Biomedical Workforce Working Group Report*; National Institutes of Health (2014). *Physician-Scientist Workforce Working Group Report.*

[27] National Institutes of Health. 2012. *Working Group on Diversity in the Biomedical Research Workforce.*

1987 to only 1.5 percent in 2014.[28] To address these challenges, Congress and NIH have introduced targeted interventions in recent years, including an expansion of the loan repayment program, pilot programs to improve or shorten physician research training, and an NIAID K99-R00 specifically for physician scientists.

Examples of recommendations in these areas that we have heard from stakeholders, or that have been proposed in the literature, and on which the Committee would be interested in the views of the community, are:

- NIH should gather demographic data and outcomes for all trainees supported through RPGs.[29]
- Universities should take action to target the postdoctoral population for improved diversity, in light of evidence that the structure of postdoctoral fellowships is deterring underrepresented populations from pursuing faculty careers.[30]
- Academic medical centers should take action to reform, centralize and better integrate medical and research postgraduate training for M.D.-Ph.D.'s.[31]

---

[28] Davila, J. R. (2016). The physician-scientist: Past trends and future directions. *Michigan Journal of Medicine*, 66-73.

[29] Ibid.

[30] Gibbs, K.D. Jr., et al. (2013).

[31] Milewicz, D. M. (2015). Rescuing the physician-scientist workforce: the time for action is now. *Journal of Clinical Investigation, 125(10)*, 3742-3747.

D

Committee Member Biographies

Ronald J. Daniels (Chair) is the 14th president of Johns Hopkins University. He holds appointments in the Department of Political Science and the Department of International Health. Before joining Johns Hopkins, he was provost and professor of law at the University of Pennsylvania and dean and James M. Tory Professor of Law of the Faculty of Law at the University of Toronto.

Daniels is a law and economics scholar whose research focuses on the intersections of law, economics, development, and public policy in areas such as corporate and securities law, social and economic regulation, and the role of law and legal institutions in promoting third-world development. Over the past several years, he has written on, and advocated regarding, the challenges confronting the American biomedical research enterprise. Recently, in concert with several of his university presidential peers, he established the Coalition for Next Generation Life Science, which commits each of the participating universities to collect and disclose data publicly on the education, training, and placement of students and postdoctoral researchers in the life sciences.

A member of the American Academy of Arts and Sciences, Daniels was also appointed to the Order of Canada in 2017 and received the Academic Leadership Award from the Carnegie Corporation in 2015.

Nancy C. Andrews was the dean of the Duke University School of Medicine and vice chancellor for academic affairs from 2007 to 2017. She is also Nanaline H. Duke Professor of Pediatrics and professor of pharmacology and cancer biology. Prior to joining Duke, Andrews was the George Richards Minot Professor of Pediatrics at Harvard Medical School, senior associate in medicine at Children's Hospital Boston, and a distinguished physician of the Dana-Farber Cancer Institute. Andrews also served as director of the Harvard-MIT M.D.-Ph.D. Program and dean for basic sciences and graduate studies at Harvard Medical School.

She was an investigator of the Howard Hughes Medical Institute for 13 years and had continuous NIH funding for her research laboratory from 1993 to 2016. Her work focused on mammalian iron homeostasis and mouse models of human diseases. She has received numerous awards and prizes for research and mentoring. She served as the 2009 President of the American Society of Clinical Investigation. Andrews was elected as a fellow of the American Association for the Advancement of Science and to membership in the National Academy of Sciences, the National Academy of Medicine, and the American Academy of Arts and Sciences. She currently serves on the Council of the National Academy of Medicine and the Board of Directors of the American Academy of Arts and Sciences, and she chairs the Board of Directors of the Burroughs Wellcome Fund. Andrews received her B.S. and M.S. degrees in molecular biophysics and biochemistry from Yale University, her Ph.D. in biology from MIT, and her M.D. from Harvard Medical School.

W. Travis Berggren joined the Salk Institute in 2007 as the founding director for the Stem Cell Research Core Facility. Berggren brought a wealth of knowledge and experience in stem cell biology to this position from the WiCell Research Institute, where he established and ran a core research program centered on mass spectrometry-based proteomic analysis of hES cells. There he worked closely with scientific director James A. Thomson and learned the "art" of hES culture from this leader in the field. Since 2010, he has taken on the additional role of senior director of scientific core facilities to provide institutional oversight for all shared scientific core resources at the institute. Berggren received a B.S. in chemistry at the University of California, San Diego and a Ph.D. in analytical chemistry from the University of Wisconsin in Madison.

Sue Biggins studies the mechanisms that ensure accurate chromosome segregation and regulation of the cell cycle. Her lab achieved the first isolation of kinetochores and has been applying structural, biophysical, and biochemical techniques to elucidate the mechanisms of kinetochore-microtubule interactions and spindle checkpoint regulation. Her lab also works on the mechanisms that ensure chromatin composition and centromere identity. Biggins obtained her Ph.D. in molecular biology from Princeton University and did postdoctoral work at the University of California, San Francisco, in Dr. Andrew Murray's lab. She joined the faculty in the Division of Basic Sciences at the Fred Hutchinson Cancer Research Center in 2000 where she is currently a full member and associate director, as well as an investigator of the Howard Hughes Medical Institute.

John Boothroyd is the associate vice provost for graduate education at Stanford University. Boothroyd is also the Burt and Marion Avery Professor of Immunology in the Department of Microbiology and Immunology at Stanford University. He received his B.Sc. from McGill University and his Ph.D. in molecular biology from Edinburgh University. Prior to joining the Stanford faculty in 1982, he worked for 3 years as a staff scientist at the Wellcome Laboratories in London, UK. In addition to his research, Boothroyd has served in an advisory role for several health-related foundations and the National Institutes of Health (NIH) as well as department chair and senior associate dean for research and training at the Stanford School of Medicine. In these various roles, Boothroyd has been heavily involved in rethinking graduate education and postdoctoral training with a focus on adapting such programs to optimally prepare a diverse population of trainees for a fast-changing job market.

David R. Burgess is a professor of biology at Boston College and a former president of SANCAS. His Cherokee great grandmother was a medicine woman, his father was a teacher and junior high school principal honored for serving minority students, and his mother was a homemaker. He was raised in New Mexico and Northern California. His current research, funded by NIH since 1977, is focused on cell division and on the science education pipeline for American Indians. He has received several awards including a Research Career Development Award from NIH and an E.E. Just Award from the American Society for Cell Biology, where he was recently elected to Council. He was recently elected fellow of the American Association for the Advancement of Science.

Burgess has served on numerous national panels, both in basic science review and on study sections whose goal is to increase the diversity of scientists. He serves on the Minority Action Committee of the American Society for Cell Biology. He has presented several keynote addresses and lectures to scientific societies, universities, and other organizations on his research and on training disparities for minorities in the sciences. He served as a member of the Advisory Committee for the NIH Office of Research on Minority Health, the Advisory Committee to the NIH Director, the NIH National Human Genome Research Institute Advisory Council, the National Science Foundation's Committee on Equal Opportunity in Science and Engineering, and the Department of Energy's Biological, Environmental Research Advisory Committee.

Kafui Dzirasa is assistant professor of psychiatry and behavioral sciences at Duke University. Dzirasa is the first African American to complete a Ph.D. in neurobiology at Duke University. His research interests focus on understanding how changes in the brain produce neurological and mental illness, and his graduate work has led to several distinctions including the Somjen Award for Most Outstanding Dissertation Thesis, the Ruth K. Broad Biomedical Research Fellowship, the UNCF•Merck Graduate Science Research Fellowship, and the Wakeman Fellowship. In 2009, Dzirasa obtained an M.D. from the Duke University School of Medicine. He was subsequently appointed as an assistant professor and house staff in the Department of Psychiatry and Behavioral Science at the Duke University School of Medicine.

Dzirasa received a Meyerhoff Scholarship at the University of Maryland Baltimore County (UMBC). He has served on the Board of Directors of the Student National Medical Association, a national organization dedicated to the eradication of health care disparities. Through his service as Chapter President, Region IV Director, and National Internal Affairs Committee Chair, Dzirasa has participated in numerous programs geared toward exposing youth to science and technology, providing health education for underserved communities, and organizing clinics to screen for chronic diseases. In 2016, he was awarded the inaugural Duke Medical Alumni Emerging Leader Award and the Presidential Early Career Award for Scientists and Engineers.

Giovanna Guerrero-Medina is the executive director of Ciencia Puerto Rico, an international network of scientists, students, and educators committed to promoting scientific outreach, education, and careers among Latinos. She is also director of the Yale Ciencia Initiative at Yale University, where she studies the impact of scientific networks such as Ciencia Puerto Rico in improving access and participation in science and works to promote diversity through the Yale Provost Office. Under her leadership, CienciaPR has become one of the largest networked communities of Hispanic scientists in the world, has secured federal and foundation grants to support diversity in science education and career development, and in 2015 received recognition as a Bright Spot in science education by the White House. Guerrero-Medina serves as principal investigator of the NIH-funded Yale Ciencia Academy, a national program to provide graduate students with opportunities for professional development, outreach, and networking. She also leads "Seeds of Success," an Amgen Foundation–supported program to promote the participation of Latina middle school girls in STEM. Guerrero-Medina has worked as head of science policy at the Van Andel Research Institute and as health science policy analyst at NIH. She has a B.A. in biology from the University of Puerto Rico, Rio Piedras and a Ph.D. in molecular and cell biology from the University of California, Berkeley, and was a 2005 Christine Mirzayan Science and Technology Policy Fellow at the National Academies of Sciences, Engineering, and Medicine.

Judith Kimble is Vilas Professor in the Department of Biochemistry at the University of Wisconsin (UW)-Madison and an investigator in the Howard Hughes Medical Institute. She graduated from the University of California, Berkeley, in 1971, worked for 2 years at the University of Copenhagen Medical School doing research and teaching histology, and then received her Ph.D. in molecular, cellular, and developmental biology from the University of Colorado, Boulder, in 1978. She was a postdoctoral fellow at the MRC Laboratory of Molecular Biology in Cambridge, England, and moved to UW-Madison as an assistant professor in 1983. Her position with HHMI began in 1994, and in 2001, she was awarded a Vilas Professorship, one of the highest honors at UW-Madison. Kimble was elected to the National Academy of Sciences and the American Academy of Arts and Sciences in 1995 and to the American Philosophical Society in 2002. She has received numerous honors and awards and has served the biomedical research community in various capacities. She served as president of both the Genetics Society of America and the Society for Developmental Biology.

Kimble's election to the Council of the National Academy of Sciences in 2008 led to membership on the Committee for Science, Engineering, Medicine, and Public Policy (COSEMPUP) and further involvement in policy. Most recently, she organized a workshop at UW Madison "Rescuing Biomedical Research from Its Systemic Flaws: Strategies and Pathways Ahead," including cross-campus discussions leading to the workshop that engaged biomedical researchers ranging from Ph.D. students and postdocs to deans and emeriti and from basic to clinical scientists.

Story Landis (NAM) was the director of the National Institute for Neurological Disorders and Stroke (NINDS) from 2003 to 2014. Landis received her undergraduate degree from Wellesley College and her Ph.D. from Harvard University. After postdoctoral work at Harvard University, she served on the faculty of its Department of Neurobiology. In 1985, she joined the faculty of Case Western Reserve University School of Medicine, where she created the Department of Neurosciences, which, under her leadership, achieved an international reputation for excellence. Throughout her research career, Landis has made fundamental contributions to the understanding of nervous system development. She has garnered many honors, is an elected fellow of the National Academy of Medicine, the Academy of Arts and Sciences, AAAS, and the American Neurological Association, and in 2002 was elected president of the Society for Neuroscience. Landis joined NINDS in 1995 as scientific director and worked to re-engineer the Institute's intramural research programs. During 1999-2000, she led the movement, together with the National Institute of Mental Health (NIMH) Scientific Director, to bring a sense of unity and common purpose to 200 neuroscience laboratories from 11 different NIH Institutes. Together with the directors of NIMH and National Institute on Aging, she co-chaired the NIH Blueprint for Neuroscience Research, a roadmap-like effort to support trans-NIH activities in the brain sciences. In 2007, Landis was named chair of the NIH Stem Cell Task Force.

Kenneth Maynard is head of Global Patient Safety Evaluation (GPSE) Compliance, Standards and Training and GPSE Business Partners Relations at Takeda Pharmaceuticals, Inc. Formerly he was an assistant professor at Harvard Medical School/Massachusetts General Hospital. His doctorate in neurobiology is from University College, London. With more than 50 scientific publications, Maynard serves on four international journals' editorial boards. He is a fellow of the American Heart Association and chair of the Professional Development Committee and councilor for the Society of Neuroscience, serves on the Executive Committee of the International Dose-Response Society, and is a consultant to the NIH Director's Program on Broadening Experiences in Scientific Training.

Gary S. McDowell is the executive director of The Future of Research, Inc. and a resident at the Manylabs open science skunkworks in San Francisco, where he works to support junior scientists advocating for changes to the scientific system. He has a B.A. and M.Sci. in chemistry and a Ph.D. in oncology, all from the University of Cambridge. Near the end of his Ph.D. study, he had a visiting scholarship at the University of Lille in France. McDowell has more than 4 years of postdoctoral experience in the United States, first at Boston Children's Hospital and Harvard Medical School and then at Tufts University. In 2015 he was part of the Future of Research team named Science Careers' "People of the Year." He is supported in his work for Future of Research by a grant from the Open Philanthropy project and in his residency at Manylabs by the Gordon and Betty Moore Foundation. He is a co-principal investigator on a National Science Foundation award addressing diversity and retention of young scientists in the science, technology, engineering, and mathematics workforce.

Jessica Polka is a visiting postdoctoral research fellow in the Department of Systems Biology at Harvard Medical School and a visiting scholar at the Whitehead Institute. Polka received her B.S. in biology from the University of North Carolina, Chapel Hill and her Ph.D. in biochemistry from the University of California, San Francisco. She is director of ASAPbio, president of the board of directors of Future of Research, and a steering committee member of Rescuing Biomedical Research. She has served as co-chair of the American Society for Cell Biology (ASCB)'s COMPASS (Committee for Postdocs and Students). Polka was a recipient of the Jane Coffin Childs Fellowship, the ASCB Beckman Coulter Distinguished Graduate Student Prize, a Genentech Graduate Fellowship, the National Science Foundation Graduate Research Fellowship Program, and the Morehead Scholarship.

Joan Y. Reede is the dean for diversity and community partnership and a professor of medicine at Harvard Medical School (HMS). Reede also holds appointments as associate professor in the Department of Social and Behavioral Sciences at the Harvard School of Public Health, and she is an assistant in health policy at Massachusetts General Hospital. Reede is responsible for the development and management of a comprehensive program that provides leadership, guidance, and support to promote the increased recruitment, retention, and advancement of underrepresented minority, women, LGBT, and faculty with disabilities at HMS. This charge includes oversight of all diversity activities at HMS as they relate to faculty, trainees, students, and staff. Reede also serves as the director of the Minority Faculty Development Program, faculty director of Community Outreach Programs at HMS, and program director of the Faculty of Diversity Program of the Harvard Catalyst/The Harvard Clinical and Translational Science Center. Reede has created and developed more than 20 programs at HMS that aim to address pipeline and leadership issues for minorities and others who are interested in careers in medicine, academic and scientific research, and the health care professions.

Reede is the recipient of numerous awards and honors including the Herbert W. Nickens Award from the American Association of Medical Colleges and the Society of General Medicine in 2005; election to the National Academy of Medicine in 2009; the 2011 Diversity Award from the Association of University Professors; and an Elizabeth Hurlock Beckman Trust Award in 2012. In 2013 she received an Exemplar STEM Award from the Urban Education Institute at North Carolina A&T University. Reede is a 2015 recipient of the Jacobi Medallion from the Mount Sinai Alumni Association and the Icahn School of Medicine.

Lana R. Skirboll is vice president of science policy at Sanofi, where she works on building academic relationships and policy issues of importance to innovation, including biosimilars, data sharing, public-private partnerships, and external innovation. She formerly served as director of science policy at NIH, where she was responsible for identifying policy issues relevant to the support and conduct of research and analyzing, recommending, and creating new policies that advance the interest of NIH. These included human subject protections, the privacy and confidentiality of research records, conflicts of interest, human embryo research, cloning and fetal tissue research, genetics, health and society, dual use research, gene therapy and nanotechnology, comparative effectiveness research, personalized medicine, among others.

Skirboll played a leadership role in NIH's organizational strategic planning and evaluation, where, for example, she developed NIH's efforts to measure and report on agency performance. She also worked with the NIH Director, Elias Zerhouni, to design and implement the "Roadmap for Medical Research." She initiated the development of a new program on return on investment to explore NIH's impact on local economies and national competitiveness. She was responsible for developing and coordinating the NIH Public-Private partnership program, which leveraged NIH investments by working with industry

Skirboll was trained in pharmacology and neuroscience. She completed her Ph.D. at Georgetown University Medical School, followed by postdoctoral work and research positions at Yale University, the Karolinska Institute (Sweden), and the National Institute of Mental Health. She is the author of more than 70 peer-reviewed scientific publications.

Paula Stephan is a professor of economics at Georgia State University. Stephan is also a research associate at the National Bureau of Economic Research. She is an American Association for the Advancement of Science fellow. In 2012, Science Careers named Stephan as their first "Person of the Year" "for especially significant and sustained contribution to the welfare of early-career scientists" during the preceding 12 months. Stephan's research interests focus on the careers of scientists and engineers and the process by which knowledge moves across institutional boundaries in the economy.

Stephan recently served on the National Research Council (NRC) Board on Higher Education and Workforce and the National Academy of Sciences committee on "The Postdoctoral Experience Revisited." She served on the NIH National Advisory General Medical Sciences Council from 2005 to 2009 and on the NSF Advisory Committee of the Social, Behavioral and Economics Program, from 2001 to 2008. She was a member of the European Commission High-Level Expert Group that authored the report *Frontier Research: The European Challenge*. She has served on several NRC committees including the committee on Dimensions, Causes, and Implications of Recent Trends in the Careers of Life Scientists; Committee on Methods of Forecasting Demand and Supply of Doctoral Scientists and Engineers; and the Committee on Policy Implications of International Graduate Students and Postdoctoral Scholars in the United States. Her research has been supported by the Alfred P. Sloan Foundation, the Andrew W. Mellow Foundation, and the National Science Foundation.

Stephan graduated from Grinnell College (Phi Beta Kappa) with a B.A. in economics and earned both her M.A. and Ph.D. in economics from the University of Michigan. She has been a visiting scholar at Katholeike Universiteit Leuven, Belgium (spring 2005); a Wertheim Fellow, Harvard University (February 2007); and an ICER fellow, Turin, Italy (fall 2009). Stephan has published numerous articles in journals such as *The American Economic Review*, *Science*, *Nature*, *The Journal of Economic Literature*, *Economic Inquiry*, *The International Economic Review*, and *Social Studies of Science*. She co-wrote with Sharon Levin *Striking the Mother Lode in Science* (Oxford University Press, 1992). Her book *How Economics Shapes Science* was published by Harvard University Press in 2012. It was translated into Korean in 2013 and is scheduled for release in Chinese later this year.

Maria Elena Zavala is a professor of biology at California State University, Northridge. Zavala holds an undergraduate degree from Pomona College and earned her Ph.D. in botany from the University of California, Berkeley. In addition to her interests in plant development, she is interested in educational equity issues, has worked to develop science curricula for K-12 teachers, has worked to improve teaching and learning in STEM, and has established and directed programs that seek to increase the number of minorities in the sciences.

Zavala's accomplishments include serving as director of the MARC/RISE and Bridges to the Doctorate Program—Maximizing Access to Research Careers, a program designed to offer mentorship, financial support, and research experience to minority students. Zavala was the first female president of the Society for Advancement of Chicanos and Native Americans in Science (SACNAS). Under her direction, SACNAS received the 2002 National Science Board Public Service Award for institutions increasing public understanding of science and engineering. She is a fellow of the American Association for the Advancement of Science and the American Society for Plant Biologists. She is a recipient of the Presidential Award of Excellence for Science, Mathematics, and Engineering Mentoring, awarded to her by President Clinton.

E

Committee Meeting Agendas

Public Agenda for the First Committee Meeting

NAS Building Room 120
2101 Constitution Avenue NW, Washington, D.C.

January 8 - January 9, 2017

Meeting Goals:
- *Introduce committee members and discuss study process*
- *Secure input from the study sponsors about the task*
- *Begin discussion of existing resources*
- *Identify key questions to address the statement of tasks*
- *Discuss plans for the study and upcoming topics and venues for subsequent committee meetings*

SUNDAY, JANUARY 8, 2017

5:00 p.m. - 6:00 p.m.   *Meeting at Hotel Lombardy*

- Chair Daniels introduces the project and the statement of tasks
- Informal discussion with invited guests summarizing previous efforts related to the initiative: Drs. Marc Kirschner and Shirley Tilghman

MONDAY, JANUARY 9, 2017

8:30 a.m. - 10:15 a.m. *Closed Session*

10:15 a.m. - 3:00 p.m. *Open Session*

10:15 a.m. - 10:30 a.m. *Break as guests arrive*

10:30 a.m. - 12:00 p.m. *Introduction and conversation with NIH*

- Dr. Michael Lauer, Deputy Director for Extramural Research at the National Institutes of Health

12:00 a.m. - 12:45 p.m. *Break*

12:45 p.m. - 2:15 p.m. *Panel discussion: Crucial Perspectives for the Next Generation of Researchers*

- *Dr. Gwyneth Card, moderator, Group Leader, Howard Hughes Medical Institute, Janelia Research Center*
- Dr. Kenneth Gibbs, Program Director, Division of Training, Workforce Development, and Diversity at the National Institute of General Medicine
- Dr. Rory Goodwin, Neurosurgery Resident, The Johns Hopkins Hospital
- Dr. Misty Heggeness, Chief of Longitudinal Research, Evaluation, and Outreach, U.S. Census Bureau

2:15 p.m. - 2:45 p.m. *Open discussion with guests*

- Committee welcomes additional input from audience members and guests

2:45 p.m. - 3:00 p.m. *Break as guests depart*

3:00 p.m. - 5:30 p.m. *Closed Session*

- Closed session for internal committee deliberations

5:30 p.m. *Meeting Adjourns*

APPENDIX E

Public Agenda for the Second Committee Meeting

NAS Building Room 120
2101 Constitution Avenue NW, Washington, D.C.

April 2 - April 3, 2017

Meeting Goals: Convene experts to:
- *Review responses to prior recommendations*
- *Consider available evidence relevant to the statement of task, including those from the NIH, university administrators, and private sector stakeholders*
- *Identify key data needs and expertise*

SUNDAY, APRIL 2, 2017

10:00 a.m. - 5:30 p.m. *Closed Session*

- Closed session for internal committee deliberations

MONDAY, APRIL 3, 2017

8:30 a.m. - 2:00 p.m. *Open Session*

8:30 a.m. - 9:15 a.m. **Presentation: Evaluating the Implementation of Previous Recommendations**

- Drs. Yasmeen Hussain and Amanda Field, Christine Mirzayan Science and Technology Policy Fellows, National Academies of Science, Engineering, and Medicine

9:15 a.m. - 11:00 a.m. **First Panel: Perspectives on Catalyzing Institutional Change to Support Early Researchers from University Administration and the NIH**

- *Dr. Nancy Andrews, moderator, Dean of the School of Medicine and Vice Chancellor for Academic Affairs, Duke University School of Medicine*
- Dr. Kay Lund, Director of the Division of Biomedical Research Workforce, Office of Extramural Research, National Institutes of Health
- Dr. Lawrence Rothblum, Chair of the Department of Cell Biology, University of Oklahoma; President of the Association of Anatomy, Cell Biology and Neurobiology Chairpersons
- Dr. Terry Magnuson, Vice Chancellor for Research, University of North Carolina at Chapel Hill

11:00 a.m. - 11:15 a.m.   *Break*

11:15 a.m. - 12:30 p.m.   **Second Panel: Creating Bridges to Research Independence through Private Sector Partnerships**

- *Dr. Lana Skirboll, moderator, Vice President of Academic and Scientific Affairs, Sanofi*
- Dr. Bahija Jallal, Executive Vice President, MedImmune
- Dr. Paul McGonigle, Director, Interdisciplinary & Career-Oriented Programs; Co-Director, Drug Discovery & Development Program, Drexel University

12:30 p.m. - 1:15 p.m.   *Break*

1:15 p.m. - 2:00 p.m.   *Open discussion with guests*

- Committee welcomes additional input from audience members and guests

2:00 p.m. - 2:15 p.m.   *Break as guests depart*

2:15 p.m. - 5:00 p.m.   *Closed Session*

- Closed session for internal committee deliberations

5:00 p.m.   *Meeting Adjourns*

Public Agenda for the Third Committee Meeting

Sanofi Auditorium
270 Albany Street, Cambridge, MA

July 12-13, 2017

WEDNESDAY, JULY 12, 2017

8:00 a.m. - 9:00 a.m.   *Closed Session*

THURSDAY JULY 13, 2017

8:00 a.m. - 8:30 a.m. *Closed Session*

8:30 a.m. - 9:00 a.m. **Overview of the NIH Next Generation Researchers Initiative**

- Kay Lund, Director of the NIH Division of Biomedical Research Workforce Programs, will brief the Committee on the latest initiatives from NIH

9:00 a.m. - 10:30 a.m. **First Panel: Perspectives from the Private Sector**

- *Jessica Polka, Ph.D., moderator, Visiting Scholar, Whitehead Institute*
- Marc Bonnefoi, DVM, Ph.D., Head of R&D France, Sanofi
- Dennis Dean, II, Ph.D., R&D Scientist, Seven Bridges Genomics
- Deborah Dunsire, MD, CEO, XTuit Pharmaceuticals
- Jim Mullen, CEO, Patheon

10:30 a.m. - 10:45 a.m. *Break*

10:45 a.m. - 12:00 p.m. **Second Panel: Perspectives from Medical Centers and Research Institutes**

- *Joan Reede, MD, MPH, MS, MBA, Moderator, Dean for Diversity and Community Partnership and Professor of Medicine, Harvard Medical School*
- Susan Baserga, MD, Ph.D., Professor of Molecular Biophysics at Biochemistry, Yale University
- Robert Blanton, MD, Assistant Professor, Molecular Cardiology Research Institute, Tufts Medical Center
- Eva Guinan, MD, Director of Translational Research, Radiation Oncology, Dana-Farber Cancer Institute
- Stephen Haggarty, Ph.D., Associate Professor of Neurology, Harvard Medical School, Director of Chemical Neurobiology Laboratory, Massachusetts General Hospital; MGH Research Institute
- Steven Hyman, MD, Distinguished Service Professor, Harvard University; Director, Stanley Center for Psychiatric Research and Core Member at the Broad Institute

12:00 p.m. - 12:30 p.m. *Open discussion with guests*

- Committee welcomes additional input from audience members and guests

12:30 p.m. - 1:15 p.m.   Break as guests depart

1:15 p.m. - 3:30 p.m.   *Closed Session*

Public Agenda for the Fourth Committee Meeting

University of California, San Francisco
Genentech Hall
600 16th Street
San Francisco, CA 94158

THURSDAY, SEPTEMBER 14, 2017

1:30 p.m. - 1:35 p.m.   **Opening Remarks by Host Keith Yamamoto**

1:30 p.m. - 3:00 p.m.   **Panel I:** *Bold Visions for the Future of Science*

- Panelists will share their vision on how changes to today's system of graduate education and early research careers can ensure a future research enterprise that fosters innovation, promotes equity and inclusion, and advances U.S. national interests.

- *Chair Alan Leshner, Ph.D., Chief Executive Officer Emeritus, American Association for the Advancement of Science*
- David Asai, Ph.D., Senior Director for Science Education, Howard Hughes Medical Institute
- Elizabeth Baca, MD, MPA, Senior Health Advisor, California Governor's Office of Planning and Research
- Michael Richey, Ph.D., Associate Technical Fellow, Learning Sciences and Engineering Education Research, The Boeing Company
- Eric Schulze, Ph.D., Senior Scientist, Memphis Meats

3:00 p.m. - 3:15 p.m.   **Break in the Atrium**

3:15 p.m. - 4:45 p.m.   **Panel II:** *Perspectives from Postdoctoral Researchers*

- Panelists will share their research on postdoctoral experiences with a focus on the implications on graduate education and early career researchers.

- *Chair Ron Daniels, President, The Johns Hopkins University*
- Marina Ramon, Ph.D., Board of Directors, National Postdoctoral Association

- Sean McConnell, Ph.D., Postdoctoral Scholar, University of Chicago
- Samantha Hindle, Ph.D., Assistant Professional Researcher, University of California San Francisco
- Paula Stephan, Ph.D., Professor of the Department of Economics, Georgia State University

4:45 p.m. - 5:15 p.m.   Open discussion with guests

- The Committee welcomes additional input from audience members and guests